OBSTETRICS AND GYNECOLOGY ADVANCES

FETAL DEVELOPMENT

STAGES OF GROWTH, MATERNAL INFLUENCES AND POTENTIAL COMPLICATIONS

OBSTETRICS AND GYNECOLOGY ADVANCES

Additional books in this series can be found on Nova's website under the Series tab.

Additional e-books in this series can be found on Nova's website under the e-book tab.

OBSTETRICS AND GYNECOLOGY ADVANCES

FETAL DEVELOPMENT

STAGES OF GROWTH, MATERNAL INFLUENCES AND POTENTIAL COMPLICATIONS

JOSIAH WILBURN
EDITOR

New York

For permission to use material from this book please contact us:
Telephone 631-231-7269; Fax 631-231-8175
Web Site: http://www.novapublishers.com

NOTICE TO THE READER

Additional color graphics may be available in the e-book version of this book.

Library of Congress Cataloging-in-Publication Data

ISBN: 978-1-63117-069-0

LCCN: 2013958102

Published by Nova Science Publishers, Inc. † New York

Contents

PREFACE

In this book the authors present current research in the study of fetal development and its stages of growth, maternal influences and potential complications. Topics discusses in this compilation include the equine fetal development, fetomaternal interaction and potential complications during pregnancy; comparative anatomy, development and functional significance of the mammalian yolk sac; influence of exercise training on e-NOS expression, nitric oxide production and mitochondrial function in the human placenta; maternal melamine and fetal development; and immunolocalization of syntaxin2 in sinusoidal endothelial cells during mouse liver development.

Chapter 1 – During gestation are implemented multiple adjustments both endocrine and metabolic adaptive aimed at maintaining maternal homeostasis. Moreover, these mechanisms ensure a uterine environment suitable for the accommodation and growth of the embryo and fetal development.

Knowledge of specific physiological events that occur during pregnancy in the mare will allow the clinician to make an assessment of the female and identify those conditions that could compromise maternal and fetal health and achieving successful pregnancy. Early conceptus development, implantation and maintenance of pregnancy are critically dependent on a precisely coordinated interaction between the conceptus and the uterine environment. Maternal recognition of pregnancy in the horse is the summation of events leading to maintenance of pregnancy; in a narrow sense, maternal recognition of pregnancy refers to the physiological process by which the lifespan of the corpus luteum is prolonged.

The horse is one of the few domestic species in which the conceptus derived pregnancy recognition signal has not been identified. In the mare, pulsatile release of $PGF2\alpha$ in systemic circulation coincides with corpus luteum regression and declining progesterone levels, indicating the probable importance of PGF2α as a luteolytic factor. The presence of the conceptus reduces pulsatile prostaglandin F2α secretion by the endometrium during early gestation in the mare. Pregnancy loss during the fetal period of gestation is a major economic concern to horse breeders. Embryonic and fetal death in mares is associated with several factors such as, oviductal and uterine environmental, luteal insufficiency, age, reproductive tract infections and abnormalities. Irregular and unbalanced nutrition and stress as well as infectious endometritis can also cause embryonic end fetal death. Pregnancy losses during late gestation could be the result of fetal illness, placental dysfunction, or maternal sickness.

High risk pregnant mares should be monitored for fetal and placental well-being. Placentitis is considered the single most significant cause of fetal loss in horses. In addition placentitis and chronic placental dysfunction contribute significantly to the delivery of premature, septic or dysmature foals that require expensive intensive care to survive. Embryo survival and the birth of a viable foal are of paramount economic importance to equine stud management. For this reason, this chapter describes the physiological events that occur after fertilization of the oocyte and during pre-and post-implantation periods of the embryo. Also, the mechanisms involved in fetal development, such as maternal, uterine, placental and hormone factors.

Chapter 2 – The yolk sac is a unique structure of vertebrates that has evolved a remarkable diversity of developmental, structural and functional characteristics. In placental mammals, it complements the chorioallantoic placenta during embryogenesis and is involved in nutrient transfer as well as hematopoiesis and erythropoiesis. The latter functions are maintained in the human, where the yolk sac is a temporary structure that participates only indirectly in fetal nutrition. The authors review what is known on relevant fetal and maternal influences, referring to the evolutionary history of the yolk sac in vertebrates and providing comparative data that includes species used as animal models for human placentation. Topics include the establishment of a yolk sac or choriovitelline placenta, including yolk sac inversion; synthesis, storage and transport of nutritional substances; cellular differentiation; vascularization; hematopoiesis and erythropoiesis. In addition, the authors review recent projects on yolk sac derived stem cells. They show that the yolk sac has maintained essential contributions to pregnancy and that it is sensitive to environmental modifications. This may help better to understand pregnancy-associated problems in the human.

Chapter 3 – A regular regimen of weight-bearing exercise throughout pregnancy has been shown to improve placental growth. The goal of this study was to determine the effects of aerobic exercise training during the second half of pregnancy on e-NOS expression, nitric oxide production and mitochondrial function in human placenta. This was a randomized, controlled clinical trial of 20 healthy primigravid women between 16 and 20 weeks' gestation. The pregnant women who were assigned to the exercise group received a supervised aerobic exercise program of 60 min sessions, three times a week. A heavy mitochondrial fraction was isolated from human placental tissue by differential centrifugation. Mitochondrial and cytosol fractions were isolated from human placental tissue by differential centrifugation. A spectro-photometric assay was used to measure NO production in cytosolic samples from placental tissue and Western Blot technique to determine e-NOS expression. Respiratory rates were determined by high resolution respirometry in placenta mitochondria from control and exercised women. Flow cytometry assays were carried out to measure mitochondrial membrane potential and superoxide levels. Combined aerobic and resistance exercise training during pregnancy leads to a 2-fold increase in eNOS expression and 4-fold increase in NO production in placental cytosol ($p=0.05$). Mitochondrial superoxide levels and hydrogen peroxide production rate were decreased by 8% and 37% respectively in the placental mitochondria of exercising women ($p=0.05$). Hydrogen peroxide production and the activity of mitochondrial respiratory complexes were also measured. Mitochondria from exercised women maintained the respiratory function and a good level of polarization. Mitochondrial O_2^- levels and H_2O_2 production rate were decreased by 6% and 26% respectively in placental mitochondria from exercised women. Activity of complex I-III of the mitochondrial respiratory chain was increased by 29% in human placental mitochondria from exercised women. Also, significant increases of 45% and 21% were observed in complexes II-III and in complex IV respectively in placenta mitochondria from exercised women. Moderate exercise can improve mitochondrial function, e-NOS expression and NO production and decrease reactive oxygen species generation at the mitochondrial respiratory chain in human placenta mitochondria.

Chapter 4 – Melamine is widely used in paint, plastic, textile and paper industries for its shrink-resistant, water-repellent, stain-repellent, and fire-retardant properties. It has made itself ill-famous by appearing in animal feeds and dairy products, affecting thousands of pets, farm animals and human infants in the early 21st century. The conventional Kjehdahl test for crude protein measurement in foodstuffs was deceived by the high-nitrogen content of melamine, disclosing the compound as an economically motivated adulteration. However, the presence of melamine in food leached from food-contacting table 'melawares' and food containers with melamine-formaldehyde coating has also been recognised as an unintentional contamination in our daily food chain. Nephrotoxicity due to the high-dose melamine intoxication from deliberate contamination have been well characterised. Histopathological findings of melamine crystal damaging the urinary system included renal tubular dilation, inflammation and carcinoma. Recent data on melamine reproductive and developmental toxicity are also identified. The maternal physiological changes during pregnancy may alter the toxicokinetic profile of melamine, which may in turn pose more serious threats to the affected mothers and their foetuses than to the non-pregnant adults. On the other hand, the developing embryo and foetal organs, not limited to kidneys, may also be vulnerable points of melamine toxicity. Prenatal exposure of melamine from the maternal intake of the contaminated pregnancy formulae and postnatal intake of adulterated infant formulae can perturb the development of the kidney, which the effect may carry on to the later stages of life. In this chapter, the reproductive and development toxicity of melamine will be addressed in details.

Chapter 5 – Syntaxin2 (epimorphin) expression was immunohistochemically examined during mouse liver development, including the adult stage, with special attention given to hepatic cell types responsible for its production. In the adult liver, nonparenchymal cells in midzonal sinusoidal regions of the lobule had strong positive signals for syntaxin2. Double immunefluorescent analyses using cell type-specific markers demonstrated that sinusoidal endothelial cells expressed syntaxin2 as cytoplasmic granules. Deposition of extracellular matrices such as types I, III and IV collagen, including those around portal and central veins, and in perisinusoidal regions, did not coimmunolocalize with the positive signal of syntaxin2.

In fetal and postnatal livers, the immunolocalization of syntaxin2 was basically similar to that in the adult liver, but its signal in the fetal liver was weak. The expression of syntaxin2 in sinusoidal endothelial cells significantly increased with postnatal liver development. Connective tissues around portal and central veins were mostly negative for syntaxin2 throughout development.

These results suggest that syntaxin2 may be involved in mature functions of sinusoidal endothelial cells, and that it may be one of their good markers in the liver. A monoclonal MC-1 antibody, which was previously shown to react with syntaxin2, stained extracellular fibers of type III collagen around portal and central veins and in the sinusoidal regions of the developing liver and adult liver. Thus, careful consideration is required when the MC-1 antibody is used for immunohistochemistry and loss-of-function experiments with the addition of the antibody. When syntaxin2 was coated on the surface of the dish in the culture of purified fetal hepatoblasts, which are hepatic progenitor cells in the fetal liver, it significantly increased their survival rate and stimulated morphogenesis of spheroid structures. This result suggests that syntaxin2 can act on hepatoblasts for their survival and morphogenesis via a paracrine loop from nonparenchymal cells.

In: Fetal Development
Editor: Josiah Wilburn

ISBN: 978-1-63117-069-0

Chapter 1

EQUINE FETAL DEVELOPMENT, FETOMATERNAL INTERACTION AND POTENTIAL COMPLICATIONS DURING PREGNANCY

***K. Satué*[1,*] *and J. C. Gardón*[2]**

[1]Department of Animal Medicine and Surgery, Cardenal Herrera University, Spain

[2]Department of Applied and Technological Sciences, Faculty of Veterinary and Experimental Sciences, Catholic University of Valencia "San Vicente Mártir", Valencia, Spain

ABSTRACT

During gestation are implemented multiple adjustments both endocrine and metabolic adaptive aimed at maintaining maternal homeostasis. Moreover, these mechanisms ensure a uterine environment suitable for the accommodation and growth of the embryo and fetal development.

Knowledge of specific physiological events that occur during pregnancy in the mare will allow the clinician to make an assessment of the female and identify those conditions that could compromise maternal

* Author for correspondence: Katy Satué. Department of Animal Medicine and Surgery. School of Veterinary Medicine, University CEU-Cardenal Herrera, C/ Tirant lo Blanc, 7, 46115 Alfara del Patriarca, Valencia, Spain. Tel: +34-961369000; Fax: +34-961-39-52-72; E-mail: ksatue@uch.ceu.es.

and fetal health and achieving successful pregnancy. Early conceptus development, implantation and maintenance of pregnancy are critically dependent on a precisely coordinated interaction between the conceptus and the uterine environment. Maternal recognition of pregnancy in the horse is the summation of events leading to maintenance of pregnancy; in a narrow sense, maternal recognition of pregnancy refers to the physiological process by which the lifespan of the corpus luteum is prolonged.

The horse is one of the few domestic species in which the conceptus derived pregnancy recognition signal has not been identified. In the mare, pulsatile release of PGF2α in systemic circulation coincides with corpus luteum regression and declining progesterone levels, indicating the probable importance of PGF2α as a luteolytic factor. The presence of the conceptus reduces pulsatile prostaglandin F2α secretion by the endometrium during early gestation in the mare. Pregnancy loss during the fetal period of gestation is a major economic concern to horse breeders. Embryonic and fetal death in mares is associated with several factors such as, oviductal and uterine environmental, luteal insufficiency, age, reproductive tract infections and abnormalities. Irregular and unbalanced nutrition and stress as well as infectious endometritis can also cause embryonic end fetal death. Pregnancy losses during late gestation could be the result of fetal illness, placental dysfunction, or maternal sickness.

High risk pregnant mares should be monitored for fetal and placental well-being. Placentitis is considered the single most significant cause of fetal loss in horses. In addition placentitis and chronic placental dysfunction contribute significantly to the delivery of premature, septic or dysmature foals that require expensive intensive care to survive. Embryo survival and the birth of a viable foal are of paramount economic importance to equine stud management. For this reason, this chapter describes the physiological events that occur after fertilization of the oocyte and during pre-and post-implantation periods of the embryo. Also, the mechanisms involved in fetal development, such as maternal, uterine, placental and hormone factors.

Keywords: Embryo, fetal development, pregnancy, risk factors, mare

1. Introduction

A normal equine pregnancy lasts almost a year. Generally 340 days is the average length of gestation but foals may be carried 3 to 4 weeks longer. A foal delivered after 310 days is considered premature. Early in gestation, between roughly day 12 and 15, the equine embryo is round and moves freely throughout the lumen of both uterine horns in response to uterine contractions. Such movement and contact between embryo and endometrium is thought to be a significant part of maternal recognition of pregnancy in horses. At approximately day 16 of gestation, a combination of an enlarged embryo and increased uterine tone leads to the embryo becoming fixed in one spot within the uterus.

This process, appropriately enough, is called fixation (Ginther, 1998). In utero foal growth and development can be affected by maternal nutrition, health, and uterine capacity (Pool-Anderson et al., 1994). The incidence of early embryonic loss (<35 days) are more common than fetal loss in subsequent pregnancy (7% versus 2.5%, Allen et al., 2007; Ezzo et al., 2011). Although most pregnancy failures occur during the embryonic period, this fact shows that fetal death is a major cause of economic loss (Jonker 2004; Krakowski et al., 2010).

Intrapartum death or stillbirth are significant (13.7%) and causes fetal abortions in late gestation. These losses are traumatic for all concerned and have a significant economic impact for the owner and horse breeding industry as a whole.

Reasons for late gestation losses are umbilical cord compromise (torsions, vascular lesions, long cords), placental compromise (placentitis, placental separation, placental abnormalities) or feto-placental infections (Givens and Marley, 2008; Vanderwall, 2008). Infectious diseases such as equine herpes virus or emerging diseases, for example, mare reproductive loss syndrome (MRLS), equine amnionitis and fetal losses (EAFL), and fescue grass toxicosis, are all associated with environmental factors and have had devastating consequences on the horse industry in the affected areas (Sebastian et al., 2008).

While 90% of all foaling proceed without intervention, the remaining 4% to 10% present a major clinical challenge. Dystocia in mares is a difficult challenge because of the vigorous nature of foaling, the potential for fatal complications, and the fact that the life of the mare and foal often lie in the hands of the practitioner. The most common cause of dystocia in mares is an abnormality in fetal positioning such as the head back position, poll lock, posterior presentation, transverse presentation, and failure of the foal to rotate into the birth posture so that the forelimbs are pushed into the birth canal upside down. Unlike cattle, absolute fetal oversize is rare in the mare (Frazer, 2011).

2. Early Aspects of Equine Embryo Development

2.1. Development in the Oviduct

After ovulation, the mare's oocyte is released through the ovulation fossa into the oviductal fimbria and progresses to the ampullary region of the oviduct where, if capacitated sperm are present, fertilization will occur (Hunter, 2012). Once fertilization occurs, the first cleavage of the equine zygote is observed 20 hours post ovulation. Subsequent cell divisions occur every 12 h, reaching the 12-36 cells stage around day 4 of pregnancy (Webel et al., 1977). From the time of fertilization, the newly formed zygote contains all of the 'information' necessary to progress through early embryonic development. It then embarks on a series of cell divisions that result in the formation of a morula (Gilbert, 2000).

The cleavage process of horse eggs is similar to that seen in other domestic mammals. Variations on the cleavage rate can affect the initial embryo development, resulting in different sized embryos of same age. Many aspects of early embryonic development in the horse are unusual or unique (Gaivão and Stout, 2012). One unusual feature of early equine embryogenesis is the polarity and opacity of the oocyte and zygote, a topic of increasing interest and practical significance in other mammals, including humans (Lechniak et al., 2008). Others include the contents of the perivitelline space, the frequently ellipsoidal shape of the cleaving egg, and the fact that the cleaving embryo acquires additional coats on the outside of its zona pellucida (Betteridge, 2000). This extrusion process of cellular material called deutoplasmolysis, is observed specially in embryos with less than 16 cells. The time taken for the cleaving embryo to traverse the oviduct, estimated to be 5.5 to 6.0 days, has been shown to be 6.0 to 6.5 days (Betteridge, 2011). The last part of the trip, through the isthmus, is accomplished relatively rapidly (Weber et al., 1996).

The reciprocal nature of the dialogue between the embryo and the mare's reproductive tract almost certainly begins immediately in the oviduct. The histochemical characteristics of the oviductal epithelium vary with reproductive status and from region to region (Raeside et al., 2004). It should be emphasized that the embryo needs always to be considered as only one partner in the physiological dialogue between it and its environment (Betteridge, 2000). Considering that, fertilized and unfertilized equine eggs are transported differentially in the mare; it seems unlikely that follicular contents influence embryo transport in the mare, as has been proposed to occur in cattle (Wijayagunawardane et al., 1999).

It should be remembered that the equine embryo spends most of its 6-day sojourn in the oviduct near the ampullary–isthmic junction of that organ (Weber et al., 1996). Functional characteristics of the oviduct manifest as effects on embryo survival evidently vary with age (Carnevale et al., 1993). The clearest evidence, however, that the oviductal epithelium affects embryo development comes from in vitro culture studies, which have demonstrated the beneficial effects of co-culture of cleaving embryos with oviductal epithelial cells (Ball and Miller, 1992). On the other hand, the equine endosalpinx cannot be absolutely essential for normal development, given that viable horse embryos can develop in the oviduct of nonpregnant ewes (Mortensen et al., 2009).

2.2. Equine Embryo Transportation to the Uterus

After fertilization and during the next 72 hours the newly formed zygote will reach the two cells, four to six cell, and eight to ten cell stage at 24, 48, and 72 hours post-ovulation, respectively. A unique characteristic of equine oviductal transport is the ability to identify and transport only developing viable embryos independently from unfertilized oocytes. The zygote and early embryo, pass all the way down the oviduct to enter the uterus through the protruberant uterotubal papilla between 144 and 158 hours after ovulation (Battut et al., 2001). The most tangible evidence of all that the embryo–oviduct interaction is reciprocal has arisen from the investigation of differential transport of fertilized and unfertilized eggs into the uterus; unless fertilized, eggs are usually retained in the oviduct. In this context, it should be noted that activation of the embryonic genome occurs while the embryo is still in the oviduct and is a gradual process at the four- to eight-cell stage (Grøndahl et al., 1993; Brinsko et al., 1995). Some experiments have shown that this is likely to involve the embryonic production of prostaglandin E2 in horses (Weber et al., 1991a,b; 1995).

2.3. Development in the Uterus

By the time the embryo enters the uterus, development has progressed to the late morula or early blastocyst stage (Betteridge, 2011). A late stage morula is essentially composed of two groups of cells; a smaller group of internal cells surrounded by a larger group of peripheral cells. Most of the descendent of the peripheral cells will take their place in the trophoblast and will not contribute to embryonic structures. Rather, the trophoblast give rises to the chorion, the outer layer of the fetal portion of the placenta. Initially, the morula does not have an internal cavity. However, during the process known as cavitation, the trophoblast cells secrete fluid to create tiny lacunae that coalesce to form a single blastocele (Gilbert, 2000).

While incipient blastocyst cavity formation has been recorded as early as 5.5 days after ovulation, day 6.5 and early day 7 blastocysts tend to show incompletely segregated inner cell mass (ICM), and it is not until late on day 7 that an equine blastocyst has a well-defined ICM and the zona pellucida begins to dehisce to reveal the newly-formed, underlying blastocyst capsule (Betteridge et al., 1982). On Day 7 after ovulation, when the ICM coalesces on one side of the blastocyst, a discontinuous layer of cells is present underlying the ICM, and isolated primitive endoderm cells can be identified lining the mural trophoblast. The Rauber□s layer is an intact flattened layer of cells overlying the epiblast cells of the ICM. However, these polar trophoblast cells are subsequently lost, and by day 10 to 12 this cell layer has disappeared completely. As early as day 8, these scattered endoderm cells unite to form a continuous layer, thereby giving rise to the bilaminar blastocyst. This formation of a primitive endoderm layer from scattered cells is unusual and diverges markedly from the pattern seen in other mammals (Enders et al., 1993).

During the same time period, a layer of endodermal cells (yolk sac endoderm/primitive endoderm) emerges from the ICM to form a second cell layer between the blastocele cavity and the trophoblast (Enders et al., 1988). Blastocyst expansion mechanisms in horses seem to differ markedly from those observed in other species; the fluid within the expanding yolk sac is markedly hypotonic (120 mosM/kg) until, after day 16, it begins to rise slowly to 250 mosM/kg at about day 22 (Betteridge, 2007).

From this moment, the yolk sac istrilaminar at the embryonic pole and bilaminar at the embryonic pole, while a simultaneous discernible thickening at the future neural folds also takes place. Within the developing mesoderm layer, blood islands form and subsequently coalesce to form a continuous vascular network and thereby establish a primitive vitelline-embryo circulatory system (Sharp, 2000). At the time of fixation (day 16-17), less than half of the yolk sac has a mesoderm layer and the developing blood vessels are concentrated around the embryo proper. By day 18, the blood vessels have anastomosed to form a network between the endoderm and trophectoderm, and adjacent to the embryo. In addition, a heart chamber and somites have now formed and the head fold is present in the mesoderm lateral to the neural tube (Ginther, 1998).

In the uterus developmental characteristics of the conceptus in the horse become especially distinct from those of other domestic species. First of all, the equine embryo, its fetal membranes and its circulatory system develop to an extraordinary extent before even the first signs of a functional yolk sac (choriovitelline) placenta at day 22 and allantochorionic placenta at about 40 days after ovulation. Second, the endodermal wall of the yolk sac is completed from cells that are unusually broadly distributed around the interior of the blastocyst, and which seem to have unusual functional characteristics (Enders et al., 1993). Third, although as in the other species the zona pellucida is shed from the blastocyst, it is replaced in the horse by a glycoprotein capsule of considerable functional importance between approximately days 7 and 21. Fourth, the encapsulated conceptus interacts with its environment during two distinct phases; it is extremely mobile until about days 16–17 and then becomes fixed at the site of eventual placentation. And fifth, the capsule maintains a spherical form for the conceptus, particularly before fixation (Sharp, 2000).

2.4. The Acellular Glycoprotein Membrane "the Capsule"

In most of the large domestic animals, the zona pellucida is the only extracellular coating to enclose the oocyte and/or developing conceptus in the period prior to implantation/true placenta formation. In the horse, however, a second acellular glycoprotein membrane known as the 'blastocyst capsule' is formed between the trophoblast and zona pellucida shortly before zona loss, and remains to envelop the developing conceptus during the second and third weeks of gestation (Stout et al., 2005). In vivo, formation of the capsule coincides with blastulation and by day 8 the capsule has reached a thickness of 1 mm (Betteridge et al., 1982).

The capsule increases progressively in thickness until at least day 11 after ovulation, but from approximately day 18 it begins to attenuate and eventually disappears completely between days 21 (Enders and Liu, 1991) and 23 of gestation (Oriol et al., 1993a). Moreover, it is likely that the presence of the tough and elastic capsule between days 6.5 and 21 to 23 is responsible for the equine conceptus maintaining a spherical shape throughout the period of maternal recognition of pregnancy (MRP), a strategy that is in marked contrast to the rapid elongation of the conceptus seen in the other large domestic species during the corresponding phase of development (Kölle et al., 2007).

The capsule is composed of a mucin-like glycoprotein, produced largely by the trophoblast (Tremoleda et al., 2003). However, the presence of mRNA from the mucin gene MUC1 in both the trophoblast and endometrium suggests that an endometrial contribution to its formation should not yet be ruled out. It is interesting that sialic acid is lost from the capsule at the time of conceptus fixation, raising the possibility of changes in charge being involved in the mechanism(s) of attachment to the endometrium (Wilsher et al., 2013). The properties of the capsule change as conceptus development proceeds. The glycosylation characteristics undergo changes at about Day 9 of pregnancy, which may be related to loss of the zona pellucida. The sialic acid content shows a marked decrease starting at day 16, which coincides with the conceptus' fixation in the uterus. It has been proposed that the capsule may have an anti-adhesive function that is regulated by the sugar side chains, i.e. the sialic acid content of the glycoproteins. By day 22.5 of pregnancy the capsule starts to disappear and is absent after day 24.5 (Oriol et al., 1993b).

2.4.1. Equine Capsule Function and Effects

The capsule is thought to provide at least three vital functions. First, the capsule is a pliable, elastic, strong structure providing protection from myometrial contractions and facilitating transuterine migration throughout the lumen before fixation (Betteridge, 1989). When equine blastocysts were capsule-denuded and transferred into its original uterus, capsule regeneration did not occur and embryos did not survive, showing that capsule formation is a stage specific event and necessary to maintain pregnancy (Stout et al., 2005). Second, it also appears to be instrumental in maintaining the conceptus in a spherical shape during early pregnancy, a feature that is very different from the elongation of other domestic embryos. Maintenance of its spherical shape and prolonged period of uterine migration are linked to suppression of PGF2α secretion by the endometrium and maternal recognition of the equine conceptus (McDowell et al., 1988). Third, the high concentration of negatively charged sialic acid residues within its constituent glycoproteins (Oriol et al., 1993a) may function to provide an anti-adhesive effect and both regulate the embryo's intrauterine movement and assist in the accumulation and uptake of endometrial gland exocrine secretions (uterine milk) (Allen and Wilsher, 2009). These secretions contain the transport proteins uterocalin (Stewart et al., 1995) and uteroglobin (McDowell et al., 1990) that are the principal source of nutrients for the still unattached conceptus during the first 40 days of pregnancy. The capsule also acts as a "mailbox" for proteins and other molecules being exchanged between the conceptus and endometrium during early pregnancy (Crossett et al., 1998; Herrler and Beier, 2000; Quinn et al., 2007).

Finally, the position of the capsule at the maternal-fetal interface suggests that is likely to play at least an indirect role in maternal-fetal signaling to establish and maintain pregnancy, for example by the temporary storage of conceptus produced insulin growth factor 1 (IGF-1) and insulin-like growth factor binding protein-3 (IGF-BP3),which is important for embryonic development (Pereira et al., 2013) and the endometrial, secreted lipocalin P19 (Stewart et al., 1995; Crosset et al., 1998). Lipocalin is foremost known as a progesterone (P_4) dependent protein secreted by the endometrium into the uterine lumen of the mare. The yolk sac wall also synthesizes and metabolizes steroids, and produces both PGF2% and PGE_2 (Betteridge, 2007; Klein and Troedsson, 2011).

At the time of fixation sialic acid is lost from the capsule. This loss does not happen if the mare is treated with PGF2α at day 14 post-ovulation (Chu et al., 1997). The loss of sialic acid in the capsule reduces the number of exposed negatively charged galactose and N-acetylgalactose residues of the major core type 1 O-glycan (Arar et al., 2007), which could be associated with changing the permeability of the capsule. It is believed that changes in charge could be involved in the mechanism(s) of conceptus attachment to the endometrium. After fixation capsule production declines until it ruptures on day 21 through enzymatic mechanisms that still remain unclear (Denker, 2000).

Legrand et al. (2001) studied the permeability of the equine capsule, using a classical freeze/thaw procedure. Researchers found the rate of dead cells after thawing was directly proportional to the capsule thickness. Embryos exhibiting a thick capsule possessed more damaged cells as a result of the freeze-thaw process, compared with embryos with little or no capsule. A negative correlation between capsule thickness and freezability of large embryos has been demonstrated in other studies and suggests that the capsule may impede penetration of cryoprotectants into the embryo proper (Legrand et al., 2002).

One of the more striking irregularities of in vitro-produced (IVP) horse embryos is the failure of normal capsule formation; even though capsular mucinlike glycoproteins are produced in vitro, they fail to coalesce into the distinct continuous capsule observed around in vivo equine embryos from the early blastocyst stage. The reason(s) for the failure of capsular glycoprotein coalescence in vitro are not known, but may involve simple dispersion of the glycoproteins into the culture medium, thereby preventing attainment of the critical concentration required for capsule assembly, or failure of hydration and cross-linking of the capsular glycoproteins in the absence of a specific uterine component(s) (Tremoleda et al., 2003). In either case, the presence of the mare's uterus appears to be essential to the process of capsule formation.

2.5. Synthesis and Secretion of Uterine Proteins and Growth Factors by the Equine Embryo

There are two basic approaches to investigating secretory products of the conceptus that are likely to be important to its interaction with the mare. The major classes of secretory products that have so far been identified include steroids, eicosanoids, proteins and peptides. Goff et al., (1993) showed that steroids is further metabolized by the endometrium and reasoned that steroids could play a role in conceptus development or the prevention of luteolysis. Raeside et al., (2009; 2012) reported that 17α-hydroxyprogesterone is the major steroid synthesized by the equine conceptus between days 7 and 14 of pregnancy. Budik et al., (2012) had shown that endoderm and trophectoderm cells from the conceptus exhibit different steroidogenic profiles in vitro, leading them to suggest that the two tissues need to act in concert if pregnancy is to proceed.

With regard to the eicosanoids, the equine conceptus continues to produce PGE_2 following its passage into the uterus, production increasing between days 11 and 15 (Vanderwall et al., 1993). The conceptus also produces PGF2α by day 14 (Watson and Sertich, 1989).

The production of proteins and peptides by the conceptus has been the subject of many investigations. McDowell et al., (1990) demonstrated that the array of proteins produced by conceptuses before day 14 differed from the array produced by older conceptuses in which a pattern characteristic of yolk sac tissue emerged. Simpson et al., (1999) have used suppression subtractive hybridization to isolate transcripts that are more abundantly expressed in day 15 than in day 12 conceptuses. They have identified cDNA clones for calcyclin (a calcium binding protein) and phospholipase A2 (involved in eicosanoid metabolism) to be differentially expressed at these times. Green et al., (1999) have identified an aspartic proteinase that is produced by the equine trophoblast as early as day 15 and which would seem to be related to the pregnancy-associated glycoproteins.

For developing embryos must alter the pattern and/or amount of PGF2α secreted by the endometrium. In cattle, sheep and pigs the antiluteolytic signal originates from the conceptus and acts on the endometrium to suppress PGF2α production. This antiluteolytic signal varies between species. In the mare the preimplantation period is long, which has a non-invasive epitheliochorial placenta that does not fully implant until day 40 post-ovulation (Bazer et al.,, 1998; Allen and Stewart, 2001).

The equine conceptus produces PGE_2 following its passage from the oviduct to the uterus, with peak production between 11 to 15 days post-ovulation (Stout and Allen, 2002). Watson and Sertich (1989) reported that 14 day old horse embryos in culture release PGF2α, PGE_2 and prostacyclin (PGI2) measured by the stable metabolite 6-keto-PGF-lα). Embryos of other species are known to produce prostaglandins (Hwang et al., 1988) and are thought to make a significant contribution to the uterine milieu in MRP. However, concentrations released by the embryos in the present study were very low compared with concentrations released by the endometrium. Merkl et al., (2010) used microarray analysis of endometrial biopsies from both non-pregnant and pregnant mares. This study revealed no detectable changes in gene regulation until day 12 post-ovulation where 332 genes were expressed higher and 42 at lower transcript levels.

Expression of these genes was validated by real-time RT-PCR. Many of these genes were known estrogen-induced genes and genes involved in regulation of estrogen signaling. Genes known to be regulated by P_4 and PGE_2 were also found. It was concluded that the target genes and pathways of conceptus-derived estrogens, P_4, and prostaglandin E2 in the maternal endometrium are involved in the establishment and maintenance of pregnancy. Other product secreted by embryo is creatine kinase (CK) enzyme. This enzyme catalyses the reversible conversion of creatine phosphate to creatine with release of the ATP. Endogenous creatine is detected in the blastocyst at a level of 0.53 pmol/embryo (Forsey et al., 2013).

2.6. Progesterone and Its Effects

P_4 supplementation has been used in animals with low post-ovulatory P_4 levels during early pregnancy and in embryo transfer protocols to create a synchronous and suitable uterine environment, allowing the embryo to develop thereby preventing luteolysis. Rambags et al., (2008) describes detection of mRNA for an equine membrane associated P_4 receptor (mPR), intracellular P_4

receptor (PR), and intracellular estrogen-β receptors (ERβ). These results suggest that progestins and estrogens may directly affect embryonic development in the horse. Therefore it is possible that maternal P_4 stimulates the conceptus to synthesize factors that play a role in maternal recognition and continued luteal function during early pregnancy.

All three of the major P_4 dependent proteins (uterocalin, uteroglobin, and uteroferrin) were detected at various levels throughout pregnancy by immunohistochemistry and histological staining of biopsies in pregnant mares (Ellenberger et al., 2008). Uterocalin secretions were highest during the peak of P_4 production by the primary corpus luteum (CL) (days 16 to 28), then declined. Uterocalin production again increased with a sharp rise when endometrial cups were formed (day 40) and again declined when cups began to degenerate. These findings agree with previous suggestions that uterocalin is a carrier protein that provides the conceptus with essential nutrients for morphogenesis and that it is the most P_4 dependent of the three proteins. Uteroferrin did not increase until day 40 when endometrial cups formed and continued throughout gestation. Formation of endometrial cups also caused a rise in serum estrogen that is thought to stimulate uteroferrin. In ovary-ectomized mares it was reported that administration of P_4 increased uterine secretions of uteroferrin and that secretion was also amplified by estrogen (Hayes et al., 2012).

Uteroglobin was detected in various low levels throughout gestation, suggesting that the P_4 /estrogen ratio may be very important in regulating uteroglobin secretion. In cattle, P_4 has been reported to affect the volume of uterine secretions and the ability to produce the luteolysis inhibitor interferon-τ (Mann et al., 2006).

Trophoblast protein-1, also known as interferon-τ (IFN-τ) is a glycoprotein secreted by the conceptus of cows and sheep between days 17 to 22 of gestation. IFN-τ is antiluteolytic and either inhibits or alters the pattern of endometrial release of PGF2α. IFN-τ also exerts antiviral and anti-proliferative activities which assist in maintaining pregnancy (Pontzer et al.,, 1988; 1991).

Maternal plasma P_4 concentrations were correlated with IFN-τ production by bovine conceptuses ($r=0.593$; $p <0.006$) (Kerbler et al., 1997). It was also noted that there was a tendency ($p=0.059$) for an increase in synthesis of IFN-τ by conceptuses from heifers treated with human chorionic gonadotropin (hCG) day 5 post-ovulation. The higher maternal P_4 via hCG treatment during early pregnancy or exogenous P_4 supplementation provides a more suitable environment for developing bovine conceptuses.

Hicks et al., (2003) investigated the link between IFN-τ and upregulation of uterine Mx gene expression in pregnant cows, gilts, and mares. The Mx gene was first characterized in sheep in response to upregulation by IFN-τ and providing immune response to viral infection in early pregnancy. Mx gene expression was upregulated in cows, gilts, and ewes during early pregnancy. There was no difference in uterine expression of the Mx gene in pregnant versus non-pregnant mares. This could be because the equine conceptus does not elongate or secrete IFN-τ during early pregnancy and fixation and maternal recognition occurs by different mechanism (Baker et al., 1991).

Monitoring serum P_4 concentrations has been a routine practice for determining phases of the estrous cycle or pregnancy in mares. Pregnancy loss occurs in 10 to 15% of mares during gestation and the majority of these losses occur during the first 40 days of pregnancy. The pregnancy is most vulnerable at this stage because the primary CL is the sole source of P_4. It has been reported that the primary CL should produce systemic blood concentrations of $P_4 > 4$ ng/ml the first 3 weeks of pregnancy (Allen, 2000: 2001a).

Papa et al., (1998) attempted to find predictive attributes of early equine pregnancy to determine possible association with early embryonic death. In this study, most embryonic loss occurred on day 19 (47%) and day 21 (29%) post-ovulation, in agreement with findings reported by Bergfelt et al. (1992). In these studies, mean embryo diameter and circulating P_4 levels did not differ between the pregnant and non-pregnant (early embryonic death) groups, suggesting that P_4 decrease is the result of and not the cause of early embryonic death in mares. The use of maternal serum P_4 concentration to estimate embryo size would be beneficial in determining the proper collection time for equine embryos destined for cryopreservation and transfer. Therefore, the objective of this study was to determine if embryo diameter was correlated with maternal serum P_4 concentration on day 7 post-ovulation. It was also reported that no correlation existed between diameter of the CL and the maintenance of pregnancy in mares. However, mean plasma estrogen concentration and embryo vesicle diameter were higher in pregnant mares, and either could be an indication of embryo viability (Scott et al., 2010).

On the other hand, coexpression of two equine genes (EqIFN-δ1 and EqIFN-δ2) coding for a protein similar to the INF family, which is the bovine, ovine and porcine signal for maternal recognition. EqIFN-δ1 and EqIFN-δ2 genes are produced during day 16 to 22 of pregnancy in the horse which coincides with the critical time of early embryonic loss in the mare (Cochet et al., 2009). The direct effects of P_4 and/or P_4 supplementation have yet to be studied on EqIFN-δ1 and EqIFN-δ2. Rambags et al., (2008) described detection of mRNA for an equine membrane-associated P_4 receptor (mPR), intracellular P_4 receptor (PR), and intracellular estrogen-β receptors (ERβ). This suggests that maternal estrogen and P_4 stimulates the conceptus to synthesize factors that may play a role in maternal recognition and continued luteal function during early pregnancy.

2.7. Embryo Mobility and Luteal Maintenance

Unlike in many other farm animals, the equine conceptus remains spherical and small in diameter. One of the most remarkable features that distinguish the equine conceptus among those of other domestic species is its remarkable prolonged mobility within the uterine lumen. Ginther used ultrasound examinations to trace the mobility of the early equine conceptus. Thus minimal movement could be observed on day 9, with an increase in mobility at day 10 resulting in maximum mobility days 11 to 14, and cessation of movement at day 16 (Ginther, 1983a; Leith and Ginther, 1984).

During the embryo-mobility phase, regardless of the side of ovulation, the embryo can be anywhere in the uterine lumen from the tips of either horn to the cervix. When first detected the embryo is frequently (60%) found in the uterine body (Leith and Ginther, 1984). Thereafter, the frequency of entries into the uterine horns increases as the embryo enters the phase of maximum mobility. The embryo enters every part of the uterine lumen and moves from one horn to another 10 to 20 times per day. Furthermore, the mobility phenomenon is an important aspect of differentiating embryos and cysts and finding and manually eliminating a member of a twin set.

Uterine contractions are needed for embryo migration, and it has been shown that uterine contractions are stronger and more frequent in early pregnant mares as compared to nonpregnant mares (Griffin and Ginther, 1990). The embryo is subjected to considerable pressure by uterine contractions during embryo mobility. So much so, that the day 13 or 14 vesicle may undergo periodic compressions (Ginther, 1989). During compression, one dimension of the previously spherical vesicle can become twice as great as the other.

The widest dimension of the compressed vesicle is in the longitudinal direction of the uterine lumen. Presumably, resiliency and elasticity of the capsule allow uterine induced distortions of the yolk-sac wall, but provide enough resistance against uterine contractions so that the embryo is moved along the uterine lumen.

Estrogen, oxytocin (OXT), PGF2α, and PGE_2 are all important in inducing myometrial contractions, and subsequently embryo mobility (Allen, 2001a), but they do not seem to be MRP signals as such. Embryo mobility itself is one of the most important factors in MRP of the horse, and there these hormones have a major role. The mobility phenomenon in mares allows the embryo to contact all parts of the uterine lining. In this manner, the relatively small spherical embryo is able to block luteolysis despite the relatively large uterus. Restricting the conceptus to a small portion of the uterus by uterine ligation prevents direct contact between the embryo and the remaining portion of the uterus and apparently results in complete or partial luteolysis although more study is needed (Griffin and Ginther, 1993). It appears that embryo mobility evolved for blocking the entire uterus in mares, whereas expansion of the trophoblast in the uterine horn on the side of the CL evolved in cattle (Franciolli et al., 2011).

The mobility of the embryo could also serve the purpose of increasing physical contact with the endometrium. Blood perfusion is increased in the vicinity of the embryo during the mobility phase (Silva et al., 2005). The mechanism of this local stimulation of vascularity is not known, but vascular stimulants produced by the embryo have been proposed. With the help of mobility, the embryo can signal its presence, and even small amounts of any substance can be effectively spread over the entire uterus to prevent PGF2α release (Katila, 2011).

Peri-implantation blastocysts of many species synthesize and secrete a variety of prostaglandins. The equine conceptus secretes PGE_2 as early as 5 days after ovulation (Weber et al., 1991a,b; 1996). Following the descent of the embryo from the oviduct into the uterine lumen, secretion of PGE_2 and of other prostaglandins, such as PGF2α and PGI2, continues. To assess the role of prostaglandins in the transuterine migration of the embryonic vesicle, Stout and Allen (2001) administered a cyclo-oxygenase inhibitor to mares between days 10 and 18 of pregnancy. The intravenous administration of flunixin meglumine resulted in a significant decrease of conceptus mobility. Flunixin meglumin is capable of inhibiting production of prostaglandins by the equine conceptus in vitro, so that it could do so if reaching the uterine lumen in high enough quantities.

On the other hand, the prostaglandins responsible for propulsion of the embryonic vesicle may be of uterine origin. Even though the uterus is not a significant source for PGF2α during early pregnancy, it may be possible that the endometrium in the immediate vicinity of the conceptus produces prostaglandin resulting in the local stimulation of uterine contractility. Given that oestrogens have been shown to increase PGF2α release by equine endometrium in vitro and in vivo (Goff et al., 1993), Stout and Allen (2001a) suggested that conceptus derived oestrogens could stimulate circumscribed release of prostaglandin from the endometrium.

Gastal et al., (1998) reported that the intrauterine administration of PGE_2 increased uterine tone and contractility, which is consistent with the contention that PGE_2 plays a role in conceptus mobility. Utilizing PGE_2-releasing simulated embryonic vesicles, Vanderwall et al., (1993) concluded that PGE_2 is unlikely to be the driving force behind the uterine transport of the latter. Allen and Stewart (2001) pointed out the apparent paradox that the driving force behind the mobility of the equine conceptus is PGF2α, the very substance that causes luteolysis and the pulsatile release of which needs to be prevented during early pregnancy. In hindsight of this paradox, these same researchers suggested that some of the early pregnancy losses occurring could be attributed to secretion of too much PGF2α by the wandering conceptus, which has the potential to enter the uterine vein and induce luteolysis.

The proposed role for the extensive migration of the equine conceptus throughout the uterine lumen is for it to secrete and distribute an unknown anti-luteolytic factor over the entire surface of the endometrium. McDowell et al., (1988) demonstrated that restriction of conceptus mobility to less than two thirds of the endometrial surface leads to pregnancy failure and that supplementation with exogenous P_4 resulted in maintenance of pregnancy, indicating that pregnancy failure was due to luteolysis with subsequent declining P_4 levels.

In the mare, the uterus exerts its luteolytic effect on the CL primarily through a systemic utero-ovarian pathway therefore necessitating the entire endometrial surface to be exposed to the conceptus-derived pregnancy recognition signal (Ginther, 1992a).

2.8. Maternal Recognition of Pregnancy

'Maternal recognition of pregnancy', is commonly used to describe the events leading to maintenance of pregnancy. In the mare, i.e. the physiological process by which the conceptus signals its presence to its dam to prolong the lifespan of the primary CL and thereby ensure a continuing supply of the P_4 on which embryonic survival and development is critically dependent differs markedly in nature to the equivalent process in other large domestic animal species (Spencer et al., 2004; Katila, 2011).

An unusual and early form of pregnancy recognition occurs in the horse, in that only developing embryos are able to initiate transport into the uterus; unfertilized ova are retained at the ampullary-isthmus junction of the oviduct. The ability of the oviduct to differentiate between unfertilized oocytes and developing embryos is based on the fact that only the latter secrete prostaglandin E_2. This hormone acts locally to relax the circular smooth muscle fibers in the oviduct wall causing the ampullary-isthmus sphincter to open, and thereby allowing the embryo to pass through and enter the uterus. The equine embryo spends nearly all of its 6-day period of oviductal development close to the ampullary-isthmic junction, whereas passage through the isthmus is rapid (hours) (Weber et al., 1991a,b; 1996). This extraordinarily prolonged period during which the equine embryo develops in the oviduct is in marked contrast to the 48 hours after which the 4-cell pig embryo (Dziuk, 1985) or the 72 hours after which the 8-cell ruminant embryo (Hafez and Hafez, 2000).

The completion of MRP (i.e., successful prolongation of the lifespan of the primary CL) is temporally coupled with a cessation of conceptus migration (fixation) on days 16-17 post-ovulation where fixation appears to be a result of the continued increase in conceptus diameter combined with a marked increase in uterine tone, which together cause the conceptus to become lodged at the base of one of the uterine horns (Ginther, 1983a,b). Early conceptus development, implantation and maintenance of pregnancy are critically dependent on a precisely coordinated interaction between the conceptus and the uterine environment. This maternal–conceptus interaction, if successful, prompts continued progestin support leading to a receptive uterine environment, which is essential for the conceptus to survive and thrive. The early conceptus signals its presence through biochemical processes that interrupt the oestrous cycle and maintain pregnancy (Stout and Allen, 2001).

The nature of the signal by which the equine embryo biochemically "notifies" the mare of its presence in her uterus and achieves the necessary luteostasis for pregnancy maintenance remains an unidentified to the present day. The equine conceptus does not produce any interferon-like protein molecules with luteostatic properties (Baker et al., 1991). However, like the young pig embryo, it does begin to secrete appreciable quantities of estrogens from as early as day 10. It has frequently been speculated that, like the pregnant pig in which the embryonic estrogens achieve luteostasis by re-directing the flow of endometrial PGF2α away from the uterine venous drainage (Bazer et al., 1998), estrogens secreted by the equine embryo may likewise constitute the MRP signal in the mare.

Mare utilizes a luteostatic or anti-luteolytic mechanism to prevent PGF2α secretion/release. At the time of expected luteolysis, PGF2α concentrations are lower in the uterine vein and uterine lumen of pregnant compared to non-pregnant mares. This shows that redirection of PGF2α into the uterine lumen to prevent it reaching the CL, like in the sow, does not happen in the mare. Another mechanism to prevent the luteolytic action of PGF2α on CL could be reduced binding to its receptor, but it has been shown thatbinding is similar in corpora lutea obtained from pregnant and non-pregnant mares (Ginther, 1992b). It has been suggested that the conceptus induces the endometrium to produce an inhibitor of PGF2α, which blocks the conversión of arachidonic acid to PGF2α (McDowell and Sharp, 2011).

PGF2α pulses stimulate OXT release from the pituitary. In the non-pregnant mare, exogenous OXT causes PGF2α release and exogenous PGF2α causes OXT release. This positive feedback is disrupted during pregnancy. Although the OXT stimulates PGF2α production, once or twice daily injections of OXT from day 8 or 9 to day 14, or subcutaneous osmotic minipumps releasing continuously small amounts of OXT prevented luteolysis in non-pregnant mares, suggesting a role for OXT receptors in MRP (Vanderwall et al., 2007). Endometrial OXT receptor concentrations are low during estrus and increase during diestrus, but more so between days 12 and 14. This increase does not take place in pregnant mares. It seems that upregulation of OXT receptors has to be inhibited during MRP. One possibility is that the conceptus produces a substance(s) that inhibits OXT receptors or interferes with the interaction of OXT with its receptor. It has also been suggested that the direction of OXT secretion is changed during MRP. Whereas in the non-pregnant mare OXT is secreted into the uterine lumen, where it acts in an autocrine way stimulating PG production, in the pregnant mare the direction could be into the myometrium to stimulate uterine contractions (McDowell and Sharp, 2011).

It is likely that estrogens produced by the conceptus are important in inducing pregnant-specific uterine proteins and in facilitating uterine contractions. The uterus-specific proteins are similar in pregnant and diestrous mares on days 12 and 14 after ovulation, but after that the secretory profile of proteins changes. Although uterine proteins are important for embryonic and placental development, their possible role in MRP is not known. Both the embryo and the endometrium produce significant quantities of insulin-like growth factor (IGF-1) which is independent of estrogen secretion (Beckelmann et al., 2013). This growth factor certainly has a role in autocrine-paracrine maternal-conceptus signaling but it is probably not an MRP signal.

Changes in gene expression around MRP are poorly understood, but researches have showed that there are genes are upregulated or downregulated between days 12 and 15 in embryos and in the endometrium, e.g. alpha-fetoprotein and pregnancy-associated glycoprotein are upregulated (McDowell and Sharp, 2011).

2.8.1. Prostaglandin F2α during the Oestrous Cycle and Early Pregnancy

Large domestic animals undergo a uterine-dependent oestrous cycle with prostaglandin F2α of uterine origin causing lysis of the CL at a species-specific time after ovulation. In the mare, pulsatile release of PGF2α, as indirectly measured via 13,14-dihydro-15-keto PGF2α (PGFM) in systemic circulation, coincides with CL regression and declining P_4 levels, indicating the probable importance of PGF2α as a luteolytic factor (Betteridge et al.,, 2012). The presence of a conceptus alters this release of prostaglandin, so that no episodic peaks of PGF2α around the expected time of luteolysis can be measured. Likewise, direct measurements of prostaglandins F (PGF) in uterine venous plasma showed that PGF concentrations at days 10 and 14 of pregnancy are lower than at the corresponding days of the oestrous cycle. Contradictory information exists regarding the amount of PGF released by endometrial tissue obtained from pregnant and non-pregnant mares in vitro. While Berglund et al., (1982) reported that endometrial tissue obtained from pregnant mares releases higher amounts of PGF, Watson and Sertich (1989) did not find a significant difference. The inhibitory effect of the equine conceptus on endometrial prostaglandin secretion can also be seen in vitro (Ealy et al., 2010). The pregnancy recognition factor produced by the equine conceptus is therefore probably primarily of antiluteolytic nature, rather than luteoprotective (i.e. inhibit the action of PGF2α) or luteotropic (i.e. support CL function). In view of this fact, it has been shown that preservation of luteal function during pregnancy in the mare is not associated with a reduction of the binding sites for PGF2α on the CL.

2.8.2. Alteration of Prostaglandin-Endoperoxide Synthase 2 (PTGS2) and Phospholipase A2 (PLA2) Expression during Early Pregnancy

During the biosynthesis of prostaglandins, cytosolic phospholipase A2 (PLA2) mobilises arachidonic acid from membrane phospholipids, which in turn is converted to prostaglandin H2 (PGH2) through the enzymatic action of either prostaglandin-endoperoxide synthase 1 or 2 (PTGS1 or PTGS2). Prostaglandin-endoperoxide synthase 1 is the constitutive isoform of the enzyme (Needleman et al., 1986), whereas PTGS2, formerly known as cyclooxygenase-2, represents the inducible isoform. The enzyme PGF2α synthase converts PGH2 into PGF2α, while PGE synthase converts PGH2 into PGE_2. PGTS1 mRNA levels remain unaltered throughout the oestrous cycle in the mare, whereas an increase in PGTS2 RNA and protein level occurs coinciding with luteolysis. In pregnant mares, such an increase in PGTS2 expression is absent, which could account for the lowered PGF2α content of the uterus during early pregnancy. The repressed transcription of PGTS2 is due to a product secreted by the conceptus, most likely the unidentified pregnancy recognition signal, as exposure of endometrial explants to conceptus-conditioned medium decreases PGTS2 mRNA abundance (Ealy et al., 2010). The expression of PLA2, which is considered a rate-limiting enzyme in the biosynthesis of prostaglandins, has recently been examined in equine endometrium during the oestrous cycle and early pregnancy (Ababneh et al., 2011). Oestrus was associated with high expression of PLA2 mRNA, while its expression decreased after ovulation. Fifteen days after ovulation, expression levels were similar between pregnant mares and cyclic mares that had not undergone functional luteolysis yet, while mares exhibiting low P_4 values on day 15 of the cycle showed higher expression of PLA2. The authors concluded that pregnancy has no effect on the expression of PLA2 and that alteration of PLA2 expression does not play a direct role in MRP. Expression and activity of PLA2 is regulated by other factors, such as post-translation modification (Klein and Troedsson, 2011).

Phosphorylation of serine residues regulates the catalytic activity of PLA2 at a post-transcriptional level and evidence exist that inhibition of endometrial PLA2 activity could occur in early pregnant ewes (Tamby et al., 1993), no such studies have been carried out in pregnant mares. It seems, overall, that alteration of PLA2 expression or regulation of PLA2 activity is not a major contributor to reduced release of prostaglandin during early pregnancy in the mare (Klein and Troedsson, 2011).

2.8.3. Role of Oxytocin and Its Receptor in Maternal Recognition of Pregnancy

The finding that in sheep peaks of OXT in peripheral plasma occur synchronously with peaks of PGFM during luteolysis has led to the notion of OXT being involved in the pulsatile release of prostaglandin from the endometrium (Fairclough et al., 1980). OXT, in general, through binding to its endometrial receptor, is a strong stimulator for uterine secretion of PGF2α (Burns et al., 1997). In turn, PGF2α is capable of stimulating release of OXT from luteal tissue (Cooke and Ahmad, 1994). Given that the CL of sheep and cattle contains large amounts of OXT, the question arises whether these elevated levels of OXT emanate from the pituitary or the CL.

The luteolytic mechanism in the mare is scarcely identified. There is evidence that OXT is integral to luteolysis in equine species. Circulating levels of OXT are highest during the mid and late luteal phase and are low during ovulation and early dioestrus. The administration of OXT during late dioestrus induces an immediate rise in the major PGF2α metabolite, PGFM. In vitro, OXT supplementation leads to an increased release of PGF2α by endometrial tissue (Ealy et al., 2010). Indirect evidence for the involvement of OXT in the regulation of luteolysis stems from the observation that systemic OXT administration initiated during the early luteal phase leads to prolongation of luteal function (Stout et al., 1999).

In the mare, OXT production has been identified in the endometrium, whereas the ovary is essentially devoid of OXT. Localization studies have confirmed the presence of OXT in luminal epithelial cells and superficial glandular cells of equine endometria (Bae and Watson, 2003). OXT mRNA expression tends to be higher during oestrus and late dioestrus than at other stages of the cycle. It has been proposed that uterine-derived PGF2α is the trigger for secretion of OXT from the pituitary during initiation of luteolysis in the mare (Vanderwall et al., 1998). What regulates the initial release of these uterine-derived PGF2α surges is unknown. Pituitary OXT then stimulates endometrial prostaglandin secretion through binding to its endometrial receptor, establishing a positive feedback loop.

OXT responsiveness is altered during pregnancy in the mare indicating that adjustment of this prostaglandin releasing mechanism contributes to maintenance of CL function during pregnancy. Fourteen days after ovulation, pregnant mares, when compared with cycling mares, respond with a diminished release of PGFM following the administration of OXT. This reduced responsiveness to OXT coincides with a decreased binding capacity of the endometrium for OXT. Likewise, pregnant mares 14 days after ovulation fail to respond with an increase in PGFM after retrieval of endometrial biopsies with OXT receptor expression being attenuated compared with cyclic mares (Sharp et al., 1997).

2.8.4. The Implication of Oestrogens as the Conceptus-Derived Pregnancy Recognition Signal

The embryo proper in early equine pregnancy has recently been shown to have a remarkable capacity for metabolism of oestrogens. High concentrations of oestrogens in yolk-sac fluid could provide substrate for local metabolism in tissues of the embryo proper and this activity could have significance for early development to development of the vasculature in the embryo at this stage (Raeside et al., 2012). Recent results by Wilsher et al. (2011) questioning the role for conceptus-derived oestrogens in MRP, as intrauterine administration of oestradiol in mineral oil did not affect the lifespan of the CL. A different experimental approach seems warranted to determine the role of oestrogens in the context of luteal maintenance.

Rather than exposing non-pregnant mares to oestradiol, the elimination of oestrogen production by the conceptus may render more valuable information with regards to this question. However, it needs to be kept in mind that local metabolism of oestradiol is significant during pregnancy. This may play an important role in the actions of the large amounts of oestradiol produced by the early equine conceptus as oestradiol may be metabolized into a biologically active product.

Furthermore, oestrogens are not the only steroid synthesized by the equine conceptus. Testosterone, androstendione, P_4, 17α-hydroxyprogesterone and 20α-hydroxyprogesterone are other steroids secreted by preimplantation conceptuses (Goff et al., 1993). Some of these steroids present precursor molecules for the synthesis of oestrogens; nevertheless, the possibility that one of these steroids is the pregnancy recognition signal has not been critically evaluated (Van Soom et al., 2011; Wilsher et al., 2011).

2.8.5. The Implication of PGE_2 as the Conceptus-Derived Pregnancy Recognition Signal

In ruminants and pigs, PGE_2 has been implicated in interfering with the process of luteolysis (Waclawik et al., 2010). In sheep and gilts, intrauterine concentrations of PGE_2 increase during pregnancy and intrauterine application of PGE_2 delays lysis of the CL. In ewes, loss of luteal mRNA for LH receptors and occupied and unoccupied LH receptors is prevented by intrauterine PGE_2 (Weems et al., 2010). Equine conceptuses secrete PGE_2 during the critical time of MRP (Stout and Allen, 2002), which may contribute to maintenance of pregnancy. Unlike in sheep, pregnancy in the horse is not associated with an increased content of PGE_2 in uterine flushings or uterine endometrial tissue (Watson and Sertich, 1989). Vanderwall et al., (1994) examined CL function in non-pregnant mares following the continuous intrauterine administration of PGE_2. Mares received either no treatment (non-pregnant control), intrauterine infusion of 240 mg PGE_2 per day (PGE_2-treated), or intrauterine infusion of vehicle (sham-treated). CL function did not differ between mares in the PGE_2-

treated group and the sham-treated group (72% vs. 36.4% prolonged luteal function). Since the incidence of sustained luteal function did not differ significantly between PGE_2- and sham-treated mares, there is still no convincing evidence in the mare for a luteotropic or antiluteolytic effect of PGE_2.

2.9. Origin of Embryonic Placental Layers

Knowledge of the layers of the yolk-sac wall and the membranes associated with transition from yolk sac to allantoic sac is required for full interpretation of the singletons, differentiating singletons from twins, distinguishing between the membranes of impinging uterine cysts and embryonic vesicles, and comprehending today's postulates on the mechanisms of embryo mobility, fixation, orientation, and twin reduction. An embryonic layer that generally is not taught in embryology courses is the capsule, which among farm animals develops only in the equine species (Silva and Ginther, 2006).

The origin of the three germ layers and their incorporation into the yolk-sac wall is diagrammed for days 9 to 15. Conversion of the single-layered wall of the blastocyst to a two-layered structure occurs upon encirclement of the blastocyst cavity by a single layer of endodermal cells. Although not studied critically, encirclement is completed by approximately day 12 (Ginther, 1992). The resulting primitive placental vesicle can be called a yolk sac, although some authors prefer to continue to call the conceptus a blastocyst until it fixes to the uterus. The endoderm of the yolk sac is continuous with the endoderm of the primitive gut (forerunner of digestive system) of the embryo proper (Gilbert, 2000; Spencer et al., 2004).

Therefore, whatever the yolk sac absorbs from the intrauterine environment becomes available to the embryo proper. Beginning growth of the mesoderm from the embryonic disc into the area between the trophoblast and the yolk sac endoderm is shown in the diagram for day 14 and by a specimen for day 15. The invasion of the mesoderm results in a three-layered wall for increasingly greater proportions of the yolk sac, as shown on the diagrams of subsequent figures. The mesoderm differentiates into supportive connective tissue and blood vessels. The day-14 vesicle is spherical even though it is freestanding, indicating that it is a turgid structure. The uterine folds are arranged longitudinally, which may favor embryo mobility (Gilbert, 2000; Spencer et al., 2004).

2.10. Luteolysis

In the absence of an embryo, the equine uterus produces a potent luteolysin (PGF2α) that travels to the ovary through the systemic circulation, in contrast with the more well-known local or unilateral route in farm ruminants. In farm species, each ovary and the major portion of the uterine tissue on that side is drained by a common vein (uteroovarian vein). In species with a local pathway (e.g., cattle), the ovarian artery is tortuous and is in close apposition to the wall of the uteroovarian vein. In a species with a systemic pathway (horses) the ovarian artery does not contact the uteroovarian vein. The presence or absence of a local uteroovarian pathway in a given species is attributable to these differences in vascular anatomy. Before the identity of the uterine luteolysin, comparisons of the uteroovarian vascular anatomy of mares (no local pathway) with that of the other farm species provided the earliest suggestion that the pathway between uterus and ovaries was venoarterial (Ginther, 1981). Experimental vascular anastomoses were used to test the hypothesis of a unilateral venoarterial pathway without assumptions on the identity of the luteolysin. The anastomoses allowed luteal regression on the hysterectomized side, whereas luteal maintenance occurred if blood was not shunted from the intact side. It is likely that the substance passing through the walls luteolithic vein and artery occurs passively (Sharp, 2000).

When an embryo is present, luteolysis must be blocked and the mechanisms by which luteolysis is abrogated in the pregnant mare are still far from being completely understood. It is best viewed as being a gradual process and clearly involves down-regulation of receptors for OXT in the endometrium so that luteolytic releases of endometrial prostaglandin F2α are prevented. Numerous P_4-dependent proteins, presumably vital to the nutrition of the conceptus, have been shown to be produced by the uterus. Of these, by far the best characterized is the lipocalin P19, which probably helps transport small, hydrophobic molecules (e.g., steroids and eicosanoids) into the yolk sac of the conceptus (Budik et al., 2012). Also many proteins found in the embryonic capsule are under investigation to determine which are of maternal origin and which come from the conceptus. Several of these are growth factors and their binding proteins (Herrler et al., 1998, 1999; Herrler and Beier, 2000).

Another hypothesis is that the antiluteolytic signal produced by the equine conceptus targets prostaglandin biosynthesis in order to prevent luteolysis. Prostaglandin G/H synthase 2 (PTGS2; also known as cyclooxygenase 2), a rate-limiting enzyme in prostaglandin synthesis, has been shown to be up-regulated at day 14-15 of the estrous cycle, but not at corresponding days in pregnant mares (Boerboom et al., 2004). Moreover, PTGS2 mRNA abundance and PGF2α concentrations have been shown to be reduced by conceptus secretions in an equine endometrial explant culture system. Therefore it has been suggested that the conceptus blocks endometrial PGF2α synthesis at least in part by repressing the induction of $PTGS_2$ expression (Ealy et al., 2010).

In addition, the equine conceptus produces a number of different secretory products during early pregnancy, including steroids as oestrogens, prostaglandins E2 and F2α (Stout and Allen, 2002), different proteins and peptides, as IGF-1 (Panzani et al., 2013), such as interferon delta, a member of the type I interferon family (Cochet et al., 2009). Moreover, the application of intrauterine devices has been demonstrated to prolong the luteal phase in the mare, indicating that a form of mechanotransduction by the migrating conceptus may prevent the endometrial cells from releasing PGF2α (Rivera del Alamo et al., 2008).

2.11. Fixation

Fixation is defined as the cessation of embryo mobility and was postulated as a mechanical phenomenon resulting from the increased dimensions of the vesicle associated with decreased luminal diameter and higher tone of the uterus. At time of fixation, less than half of the yolk-sac wall has developed a third layer (mesoderm), and blood vessels have begun to develop in the mesoderm near the embryo proper (Ginther, 1992a). A cavity, the exocoelom, forms within the mesoderm near the embryo proper, dividing the mesoderm into two layers.

Folds of ectoderm and mesoderm begin to pass over the embryo proper and will give rise to the amnion. The membrane consisting of ectoderm and mesoderm is called the chorion. Fixation occurs on mean days 15 in ponies and 16 in horses near a flexure in the caudal portion of one of the uterine horns. It has been postulated that fixation occurs at this site despite continuing uterine contractions because the flexure is the greatest mobility (Griffin and Ginther, 1990; Gastal et al., 1996).

The equine uterus is flaccid during and immediately after estrus as shown for day 3, increases in tone until mid-diestrus, decreases in tone until day 10 or 11, and then, if the mare is pregnant, gradually increases in tone and becomes turgid (Bonafos et al., 1994) as shown for day 16. The increase in uterine tone is associated with a decrease in uterine diameter (Griffin and Ginther, 1991a; Bergfelt and Ginther, 1996) and continues until days 25 to 30 as shown for day

30 (Bonafos et al., 1994). The gradually increasing uterine tone and decreasing uterine diameter together with increasing conceptus diameter apparently combine to result in fixation of the conceptus (Ginther, 1995). The conceptus distributes a tone-stimulating substance during embryo mobility; uterine ligation studies demonstrated that tone was greater in uterine horns exposed to the embryo and estradiol may contribute to tone stimulation (Griffin and Ginther, 1993). Gastal et al., (1998) suggest that PGE_2, produced by the embryo plays a role in both stimulating uterine contractions and increasing uterine tone during the embryo-mobility phase. A continuing P_4 source is necessary for embryo mobility and fixation. When luteolysis occurs after fixation, the uterus loses its turgidity, and the embryo leaves the site of fixation. Sometimes the embryonic heart is still beating after the embryo leaves the fixation site; embryonic death, however, is imminent (Willmann et al., 2011).

2.12. Orientation

Orientation is defined as rotation of the embryonic vesicle so that the embryo proper is on the ventral aspect of the yolk sac.The importance of orientation at this time will become clear in the discussions on the transition between yolk sac and allantoic sac and formation of the umbilical cord. However, the mobile prefixation vesicle probably rotates, and the embryonic disc can be anywhere on the circumference at this time. In this regard, simulated embryonic vesicles tend to roll when responding to uterine contractions.

The yolk sac is three-layered and vascularized at the embryonic pole and two-layered at the opposite pole. The islands of blood cells that developed in the mesoderm of the three-layered portion have coalesced to form a continuous vascular network. It has been postulated that orientation occurs between the time of fixation and the appearance of the irregular shapes (Ginther, 1985a).

Three factors are believed to interact during orientation (Ginther, 1983a,b; 1985b):

1. Thick (three-layered) and thin (two-layered) portions of the yolk-sac wall;
2. Asymmetrical encroachment from thickening of the upper turgid uterine wall on each side of the mesometrial attachment;

3. The massaging action of uterine contractions. The interaction of these factors results in the thickest portion of the yolk-sac wall (embryonic pole) rotating to a ventral position (antimesometrial).

It is not clear, however, whether the localized thickening of the endometrium adjacent to the thin-walled portion of the yolk sac occurs before, during, or after orientation; the cause of the thickening has not been determined. The orientation hypothesis is compatible with six reported cases of disorientation associated with a flaccid uterus or the presence of twin vesicles at the postulated time of orientation (Ginther, 1985a; 1995) Once fixation and orientation are established, increasing horn turgidity, cranial and caudal to the vesicle, prevents the vesicle from dislodging longitudinally in the uterine lumen. The orientated position, as viewed in cross-section, apparently is aided by adhesiveness and cross-ridging of the endometrial folds. Later, after loss of the capsule on day 21, a ridge of trophoblast indents the endometrium and may further anchor the vesicle and help prevent rotation (Enders and Liu, 1991).

2.13. Endometrial Cups

The formation of endometrial cups is first manifests between days 38 and 40 as a series of small, pale, slightly raised plaques on the surface of the endometrium arranged in a circle around the conceptus at the base of the gravid uterine horn. Formation of the endometrial cups involves restructuring of intermingling placental and maternal cells. The cups represent intricate microphysical and chemical interactions between the uterus and conceptus (Wooding et al., 2001). A band of specialized trophoblastic cells (chorionic girdle) develops over days 28 to 355 and encircles the conceptus in the avascular area of the chorion at the junction of the yolk sac and allantoic sac (Stewart et al., 1995). The mature chorionic girdle at days 35 or 36 is a 9-mm wide band that attaches to the endometrial epithelium. A small proportion of the girdle cells successfully invade the maternal tissue to form the endocrine cells of the cups (Enders and Liu, 1991).

Although the cups develop entirely within the maternal endometrium and show no physical attachment to the overlying allantochorion, they are, in fact, fetal in origin. The morphogenesis of the cups, as described by English workers is depicted. Girdle-cell invasion involves amoeboid-like phagocytosis and digestion of the epithelial cells of the uterus, followed by migration into the endometrium. The differentiated cup cells produce equine chorionic gonadotropin (eCG). The large fetal endometrial cup cells are the source of the high concentrations of eCG that circulate in the blood of pregnant equids between days 40 and 120 of gestation (Allen, 1969a,b). This high molecular weight (72 KDa) glycoprotein expresses both FSH- and LH-like biological activities in a ratio of approximately 1.4:1, and it ovulates or luteinizes (without ovulation) dominant ovarian follicles that develop during the first half of pregnancy by continuation of surges in pituitary FSH concentrations in maternal blood. Thus, secondary corpora lutea begin to form from the time of first appearance of eCG and this, in turn, results in rises in maternal serum P_4 concentrations.

The irregular shape and sizes (a few millimeters to several centimeters) of individual cups is attributable to variation in girdle-cell contact across the irregular topography of the endometrial folds. Similar weight of the cups (about 10 g) in pony and horse mares is attributable to a similar diameter of the conceptus at day 36 and accounts, at least in part, for the higher eCG concentrations in ponies because of the smaller blood volume (Ginther, 1992b).

Each cup represents a discreet package of adjacent cells with different genotypes (maternal and fetal). They are in effect, fetal allografts. The fetal antigens are foreign to the mare, resulting in an influx of immune lymphocytes that is the most striking known example in any species of a cell mediated immune response to pregnancy. In this regard, the immunologic aspects of the endometrial cups may be the most intensively researched aspect of mare reproductive biology. The lymphocytes have the potential of destroying the foreign tissue. It appears that the cups initially defend against the lymphocytic attack, but eventually the defensive mechanism is overcome and apparent lymphocytemediated demise of the cups begins (Allen and Wilsher, 2009).

At the approximate time that eCG appears in the blood, the primary CL begins to resurge in size (Bergfelt et al., 1989) increase its productivity of P_4, and initiate the production of estradiol (second luteal response to pregnancy. Formation of supplementary corpora lutea is also closely and temporally related to circulating eCG concentration (third luteal response to pregnancy. The luteal source of P_4 and estrogen from eCG stimulation declines as the fetoplacental source inclines, suggesting that a role of eCG is to stimulate a temporary source of these steroids until the fetoplacental source is adequate. Another suggested role of the cups is to prepare immunologically the uterine environment for the later intricate and intimate microcotyledonary attachment of the allantochorionic placenta to the uterine lining (Ginther, 1992a).

3. The Fetal Stage

3.1. Development of the Fetus, Placentation and Steroidogenesis

By the beginning of the fetal stage (day 40), the amnion is vascularized and the pontine flexure of the embryo stage is gone. The fetus has arrived at the pole opposite the pole of the orientated embryo proper. Replacement of the yolk-sac placenta by the allantochorionic placenta is nearly complete. The membranes and associated vessels separating the yolk sac and allantoic sac are coming together and will form the umbilical cord.

The umbilical cord lengthens so that the fetal-amniotic unit reaches the lower wall or ventral aspect of the allantoic sac by day 48 (Ginther, 1993). Furthermore, the site of the allantochorionic attachment of the umbilical cord throughout pregnancy identifies the horn and site where embryo fixation occurred.

Placentation commence around day 40 to 42 and within only a day or two after invasion of the maternal endometrium by the chorionic girdle cells that will initiate endometrial cup formation, the non-invasive trophoblast cells of the allantochorion at last begin to establish a microvillous attachment to the luminal epithelial cells of the endometrium. The allantochorion starts to elongate steadily, and at the feto-maternal interface, blunt finger-like villi of allantochorion interdigitate with thin, more elongated and branching outgrowths from the surface of the endometrium. Beyond day 60, both the maternal and fetal components of this steadily deepening interdigitation begin to become extensively branched so that, by around day 120, the fundamental haemotrophic exchange unit of the allantochorionic placenta, the micro-placentome, is well formed, and these maternofetal interdigitatory structures cover the entire maternal surface of the diffuse placenta (Bracher et al., 1996).

In addition to the extensive development of the microplacentomes and their haemotrophic exchange mechanisms, the long, multibranched endometrial glands remain functional throughout gestation and release their protein-rich exocrine secretions into well-defined spaces, termed areolae, between adjoining microplacentomes. A healthy and extensive micro-cotyledonary placenta attached to a healthy and fully functional endometrium is a prerequisite for a successful pregnancy in the mare. Any diminution in this vast area of intimate fetomaternal contact will lead to a certain degree of runting and weakness in the newborn foal or may cause embryonic death early in gestation or abortion later in pregnancy (Marenzoni et al., 2012). Twinning is a classic example of this phenomenon since the allantochorions of the two conceptuses compete for the limited surface area of endometrium to which they may attach.

Another unusual phenomenon of equine pregnancy is the enormous growth and subsequent regression of the fetal gonads during the second half of gestation. About day 80 in both male and female fetuses, the gonads begin to enlarge steadily until they reach a maximum size and combined weight of approximately 350 g between days 230 and 260. The gonads begin to shrink after day 270 and have reduced in size and appearance by day 336 to the small, relatively insignificant structures one anticipates of neonatal gonads in other large domestic animals.

In close parallel with this event, maternal serum estrogen concentrations rise steadily to reach peak values as high as 400 ng/ml between days 190 and 250 and decline thereafter to baseline values at term. The biological significance of the estrogens secreted by the equine feto-placental unit are not well understood although they may play a role in regulating both uterine and placental blood flow, as has been shown to be the case in the pregnant ewe (Pupkin et al., 1975), and in the synthesis and storage of prostaglandin precursors in the endometrium and myometrium.

Feto-placental production of P_4 and other C-21 progestagens in the pregnant mare differs significantly from estrogens. The placenta begins to produce appreciable quantities of progestagens from around day 70. Furthermore, a definite rise in maternal plasma progestagen concentrations, which is more pronounced in Thoroughbred than Pony mares (Hamon et al., 1991), occurs during the last 4 to 6 weeks of gestation (Holtan et al., 1991) and is followed by a sharp decline in values only during the immediate preparturient period.

The source of this unusual, late-gestation rise in plasma progestagen concentrations in pregnant mares and its biological significance in fetal maturation and parturition has aroused much speculation and investigation over the past two decades (Rossdale and Silver, 1982; Rossdale et al., 1992). Thorburn (1993) and Chavatte et al. (1997) speculated that the pregnenelone required for this additional progestagen synthesis by the placenta is secreted by the steadily enlarging fetal adrenal gland. A lack of 17α-hydroxylase activity in the adrenal cortex at this stage prevents pregnenelone from being metabolized to cortisol, and it instead passes to the placenta where it is converted into 5α-reduced pregnanes due to the persisting high levels of 5α-reductase enzyme in placental tissue. Then these products enter the fetal and maternal circulations (Abd-Elnaeim et al., 2009).

3.2. Fetal Mobility

During months 2 to 4, the length of the umbilical cord and the volume-ratio of allantoic fluid to fetal mass increases considerably. The fetus moves about within the relatively large pool, tied only by a long lifeline "the umbilical cord". Episodes of fetal activity, such as neck arching and limb thrusts, propel the fetus off the inner wall of the allantochorion and into the pool of allantoic fluid. Sometimes the fetal-amniotic unit is enclosed in a uterine horn and then appears to be forced through a constriction into a dilated portion. The fetus changes direction, recumbence, and location with great vigor and seemingly practices the neuromuscular coordination that it will need during independent life, including those required for limb action, head shaking, nursing, and chewing. For example, the fetus changed presentation a mean of five times/hour during month 3 (Griffin and Ginther, 1991). Because of rapid fetal enlargement, the relative volume of the placental pool decreases over months 4 to 9, and the meanderings of the fetus diminish, but the in-place activity remains.

The extensive mobility of the fetus within the allantoic sac was discovered by transcervical endoscopy and confirmed by transrectal ultrasonography. Fetal mobility is sometimes attributable to extraneous movements (mare, intestine), but mobility depends primarily on the fetus injections of succinylcholine, a neuromuscular blocker, into the fetus reduced the number of changes in location and presentation by five-fold. The phenomena of mobility and activity complicate attempts to ultrasonically examine the fetus, such as during a search for twins or the diagnosis of fetal gender (Griffin and Ginther, 1991; 1993).

The orientation of the uterine horns to the uterine body changes dramatically as pregnancy advances (Ginther et al., 1994). Initially, the horns point cranially and dorsally. As the conceptus enlarges, the uterus sinks further into the intestinal viscera and the horns gradually assume a perpendicular orientation. The horns are approximately perpendicular to the upper-cranial aspect of the uterine body by months 6 and 7. As the fetus enlarges, the dome-like cranial portion of the uterine body and adjacent caudal limb horn move further cranially, and the dorsal surface of the horns (mesometrial attachment) move increasingly closer to the dorsal surface of the uterine body. Thus, by month 11 the mesometrial surface of the limb horn is often in close apposition with the mesometrial surface of the uterine body; the horn lays on the surface of the uterine body with the tip of the horn directed toward the cervix.

The tips of the horns and ovaries are attached by relatively short ligaments, accounting for the change in orientation of the horns as the uterine-body enlarges (Ginther, 1993).

4. MATERNAL INFLUENCES AND POTENTIAL COMPLICATIONS

4.1. Fetomaternal Interactions and Influences during Equine Pregnancy

4.1.1. Luteal Deficiency and Embryo Mortality in the Mare

The mare has evolved an even more unusual system with regard to the roles of the ovaries and placenta in supplying the P_4 needs of pregnancy. Mare s primary CL, which develops from the ovulation that led to the pregnancy, persists beyond its normal cyclical lifespan (15-16 days) due to the actions of a hitherto undefined MRP factor secreted by the spherical and mobile conceptus. Having escaped luteolysis during day 14-16, the equine CL hangs on and persists in the ovary as in other species but it declines steadily in its P_4 output over the next 18-20 days to the extent that peripheral plasma P_4 concentrations in most mares fall from a dioestrous peak of 12-20 ng/ml around days 5-10 after ovulation to values as low as 3-5 ng/ml by day 35. The strong impression is gained that the primary CL, once saved from destruction at day 14-16, persist in the ovaries without any form of luteotrophic stimulus from then until day 38-40 when it does indeed receive support in the form of equine chorionic gonadotrophin (eCG) (Allen, 2001a).

Coincidentally with this period of `indifference' of the primary CL, the maternal ovaries continue to show 10-12 day waves of follicular growth, just as in the oestrous cycle, that are clearly stimulated by the continuation of the light-driven 10-12 releases of pituitary follicle-stimulating hormone (FSH). However, none of these follicles reach full maturity and ovulate because of suppression of pituitary luteinizing hormone (LH) release by the negative feedback effects of the continuously high P_4 concentrations. Then, between days 38 and 40 in the great majority of pregnant mares, and closely coincidental with the onset of eCG secretion by the endometrial cups, one of these secondary follicles does ovulate in response to the LH-like biological activity of the chorionic gonadotrophin. Plasma P_4 concentrations rise sharply, and thereafter at roughly 10-15 intervals, further accessory ovulations occur by the same process as the LH-like activity of the relatively huge concentrations of eCG in maternal blood inducing maturation and ovulation of the most advanced of the next wave of follicles developing in response to the continuing releases of pituitary FSH (Allen, 2001a).

During the period of expansion of the allantochorion and its development of the mature microcotyledons between days 40 and 120 of gestation, the trophoblast cells acquire a comprehensive repertoire of hormone synthetic capabilities. These include eCG from the invasive endometrial cups from day 38-40 relaxin from around day 45-50 (Klonisch et al., 1997), the phenolic oestrogens, oestrone and oestradiol and the equine-specific ring b unsaturated oestrogens, equilin and equilenin from around day 70-80. Thus, between days 70 and 150 of gestation in the mare, peripheral plasma concentrations of P_4 and related progestagens represent a mixture of ovarian P_4 secreted by the declining primary and secondary CL and placental progestagens secreted by the enlarging allantochorion. Holtan et al., (1975) in a study concluded that the placenta had become suficiently mature to take over entirely the role of "P_4 provider" between days 70 and 100. Therefore it seems reasonable to suggest that this time coincides closely with the expansion of the allantochorion to the tip of the non-gravid horn so that the whole area of lumenal epithelium is attached to trophoblast cells of the allantochorion. From this time onwards the myometrial and endometrial tissues of the uterus will receive placental progestagens by direct diffusion from the closely adhered placenta so that the P_4 still being secreted by the multiple CL in the ovaries will become somewhat superfluous.

When all the ovarian CL finally regresses in midgestation, maternal plasma progestagen concentrations remain low for the next 4-5 months. The main supply tissue, the placenta, is in direct and intimate contact with the principal target tissue, the endometrium, over the entire area of both organs, which means that the progestagens measured in peripheral blood represent overspill and/or metabolites and the concentration bears little relationship to what actually is happening in the uterus (Allen, 2001a). During the last 4-6 weeks of gestation maternal blood progestagen concentrations rise again quite steeply by 24-48 h before foaling, after which they fall sharply.

In view of the complexity and the interdependence of these various sources of P_4 in the pregnant mare the question arises as to whether an abnormality or inadequacy of function of any of the sources occurs commonly and whether it creates enough of a deficiency in P_4 production to cause fetal death and abortion (Allen 2001a,b). Looking at the first 40 days of gestation, when the P_4 is supplied exclusively by the prolonged primary CL, a sudden and unexpected failure of that structure, caused by an untoward release of PGF2α, would obviously cause pregnancy loss if for no other reason than that the resulting relaxation of the cervix and the increase in rhythmical contractility of the increasingly oestrogen-dominated myometrium would eventually result in expulsion of the already dying conceptus from the uterus (Newcombe, 2000). Indeed, this prolonged pregnancy CL becomes susceptible to luteolytic destruction after day 18 because of a renewed appearance of the previously suppressed endometrial OXT receptors from around this time (Stout and Allen, 2001).

PGF2α release stimulated by endotoxaemia of gastrointestinal origin, or by injection of endotoxin, will cause luteolysis and pregnancy loss during the first 40 days of gestation in the mare, but not after this time, due to the strong luteotrophic support of eCG for the secondary CL. Furthermore, these endotoxaemia-induced abortions can be prevented by the simultaneous administration of exogenous progestagen and/or the prostaglandin synthetase inhibitor, flumixin meglumine. Thus, it seems clear that the primary CL of pregnancy in the mare, which is the sole source of P_4 during the first 40 days of gestation, is a `prolonged CL' that escaped destruction around day 14-16 by suppression of PGF2α release at that time. It has no luteotrophic support from then until the beginning of eCG secretions at day 38-40 and it appears to be highly susceptible to luteolytic mechanisms in this period. Furthermore, with the upregulation of endometrial OXT receptors that has been demonstrated in the pregnant mare from day 18 after ovulation the uterus clearly remains geared up and ready to trigger the luteolytic pathway should it receive an appropriate stimulus. With this delicate situation in place until secondary luteal development after day 40, and with a conceptus that actively secretes both PGE_2 and PGF2α to ensure its propulsion throughout the uterine lumen during days 6-17 after ovulation it could seem reasonable to expect that some form of luteal inadequacy, either by the failure of the primary CL to develop properly, or to suffer untoward luteolysis triggered by colic or any other source of endotoxin, would be a common cause of early pregnancy failure in the mare (Stout and Allen, 2001).

Morris and Allen (2002) determined that as many as 63% of all the pregnancy losses recorded throughout gestation in this cohort of mares occurred between days 15 and 45 after ovulation. However, early fetal death in the mare could have many other causes, including: (1) accidental misalliance of male and female chromosomes at the time of fertilization; (2) incipient low-grade bacterial or fungal endometritis that colonizes and destroys the young conceptus; and (3) age-related degenerative changes in the endometrium (endometrosis) causing `nesting' of the. The necessity of adequate supplies of uterine proteins during this very early period is perhaps best illustrated by the very high rate (> 50%) of resorption, between days 18 and 25 after ovulation, of one of twin conceptuses that become `fixed' together around day 16 in the base of the same uterine horn. Thus, during the first 40 days of pregnancy in the mare, a fairly high rate (‹10%) of pregnancy failure occurs and the reproductive tract seems primed, ready to initiate luteolysis at a stroke should even the vaguest of stimuli pull the luteolytic trigger.

Although the primary CL is clearly vulnerable to untoward luteolysis during the first 40 days of gestation this seems to happen rarely (Irvine et al., 1990) and, indeed, clinical stud veterinary experience tells that in the great majority of mares which do undergo early embryonic death and resorption in the early period, luteal function persists and the mare requires treatment with $PGF2\alpha$ or one of its analogues to induce her to return to oestrus (Newcombe, 2000). When the secondary CLs begin to develop from day 40 onwards, eCG exerts a powerful luteotrophic effect upon them and clinical experience again relates that they can be very resistant to even repeated treatments with prostaglandin (Allen, 2001a). Thus, it is difficult to conceive of the situation in a mare whereby, in the face of even lower-than-normal levels of eCG produced by functioning endometrial cups luteal deficiency could occur to the point whereby insuficient P_4 was being secreted by the ovaries to maintain the pregnancy state.

Despite this overwhelming lack of both theoretical and actual evidence that P_4 deficiency from any quarter is a significant underlying cause of pregnancy loss in the mare, and even in the face of the recent evidence of McKinnon et al., (2000) that most commercially available preparations of synthetic progestagens commonly given to pregnant mares show no biological activity in the horse, kilograms of progestagen are poured or injected into thousands of pregnant mares annually throughout at least the Western world. There really exists an urgent need for some properly controlled trials to either justify or debunk such practice.

4.1.2. Role of the Embryonic Vesicle and Progesterone in Embryonic Loss in Mares

Many factors have been associated with spontaneous embryonic loss in mares (Ball, 1988). Small embryonic vesicles during the embryo mobility phase (days 11-15) are indicators of increased probability of impending loss, even though growth rate is usually similar to that of normal-sized vesicles. Embryos that are lost are more frequently located in the uterine body during the mobility phase. This was due to the small diameter, since normal vesicles of a corresponding diameter (days 9-11) are morefrequently found in the uterine body (Ginther, 1992b).

Reduced concentrations of P_4 have been associated with spontaneous embryonic loss in mares and could involve (i) induced luteolysis due to endometritis, (ii) failure of the conceptus to block luteolysis, or (iii) primary luteal insufficiency. After spontaneous embryonic loss, the primary CL was maintained more often when loss occurred after day 20 than when loss occurred before day 20. However, the roles of the embryonic vesicle and circulating P_4 concentrations in association with embryonic loss have not been described adequately in relation to the day of loss. It has been reported that resurgence of the primary CL (increase in size and P_4 production) occurs between days 35 and 40 of pregnancy and is attributable to the release of eCG into the circulation. Presumably, the CL that was subsequently maintained in mares with embryonic loss would not increase in size provided loss occurred before invasion of trophoblastic cells into the endometrium with resulting production of eCG (Bergfelt et al., 1992).

Formation of an embryonic vesicle without development of the inner cell mass or embryo has been reported anecdotally. Abnormal embryonic development in mares, characterized by formation of an embryonic vesicle without an embryo, results when formation or development of the inner cell mass or embryo is disrupted. At the blastocyst stage of development (between days 7 and 10 after ovulation), the blastocoel is lined by a single layer of cells of ectodermal origin termed the trophoblast. Most of the trophoblast will contribute to the formation of the placenta. When the inner cell mass fails to form or develop, the trophoblast can apparently continue to grow (ie, increase in diameter), but it cannot complete normal development (Vanderwall et al.,, 2000). Development of an embryonic vesicle without an inner cell mass or embryo has important implications for clinical management of early pregnancy in mares. Transrectal ultrasonography can generally be used to identify the embryo within the embryotic vesicle as early as day 20 after ovulation, whereas the embryonic heartbeat is generally detectable by day 24 or 25 (Ginther, 1986). Therefore, to identify this specific type of abnormal embryonic development, mares should be examined on day 25 after ovulation for detection of the embryo and embryonic heartbeat. For mares in which the embryo is not detected on day 25, additional examinations should be performed every 1 to 3 days until day 30.

In normal conceptuses, it is possible, although rare, that the embryo or embryonic heartbeat may not be readily identified until day 30. However, the embryo and embryonic heartbeat have always been detectable by day 30. Therefore, if the embryo is not visible by day 30, the conceptus should be identified as abnormal. Because 5 of 7 abnormal embryonic vesicles were undersized in the mares reported here, small conceptuses should be monitored closely. When an embryonic vesicle without an embryo is identified, 2 management options exist. 1.- Conservative management consists of monitoring the abnormal conceptus by use of transrectal ultrasonography and allowing the mare to naturally eliminate it. 2.- Active management consists of terminating the abnormal pregnancy by administering a luteolytic dose of PGF2α alone or in combination with manual transrectal reduction of the conceptus.

Although PGF2α treatment alone will eliminate a conceptus at that stage of gestation, on average, complete loss of the conceptus requires more than one week when PGF2α is administered on day 30. By disrupting the embryonic vesicle, manual reduction may hasten complete elimination of the conceptus, although the amount of time that conceptus fragments persist after manual reduction is unknown (Vanderwall et al., 2000).

4.1.3. The Pattern of Embryonic Fixation and Its Relatioship to Pregnancy Loss in Mares

Embryo survival and the birth of a viable foal are of paramount economic importance to equine stud management. Fixation of the equine embryonic vesicle (EV) occurs at around day 16 post-ovulation, when the period of embryo mobility ceases. At this stage the embryo permanently attaches to the uterine endometrium, often at either of the corpus–cornual junctions (Carnevale and Ginther, 1992). The effect of side of EV fixation on pregnancy loss in the mare has also received little attention to date, although some work has used transrectal palpation records in attempts to account for embryonic and early fetal loss or general fetal loss occurring between day 42 and foaling (Gilbert and Marlow, 1992).

Mare age had no effect on the side of EV fixation; however, mare reproductive status did, EV□s fixed more frequently in the right uterine horn in maiden and barren mares. The proposed underlying mechanism for EV fixation in mares involves a decrease in embryo mobility within the uterus. This may in part be attributed to the combined effects of the growing conceptus and increasing uterine tone as well as declining embryonic prostaglandin production which reduces uterine contractility (Griffin and

Ginther, 1990). The sharp curvature / flexure of the corpus–cornual junction further reduce embryo mobility in this area and so facilitates EV fixation (Gastal et al., 1996).

The equine uterus involutes rapidly after foaling, both physically and histopathologically. By the time an embryo, resulting from a foal heat breeding enters the uterus, endometrial recovery and fluid clearance may still be incomplete in the horn from which the mare delivered her mostrecent foal (previously gravid horn) which takes relatively more time to involute than the previously non-gravid horn. This difference probably results in the previously non-gravid horn being able to provide the greatest resistance to embryo movement and a more conducive environment for embryo development (Sharma et al., 2010). EV fixed in the horn ipsilateral to the previously gravid horn in lactating mares is significantly more likely to be lost during the embryonic period (Davies Morel et al., 2009). It suggests that despite functional uterine involution, it is the parity related endometrial degenerative changes which are probably more pronounced in the ipsilateral horn and may account for more pregnancy losses particularly during the embryonic phase. The observation of a higher tendency for overall pregnancy losses in the ipsilateral horn is a reflection of the inability of the ipsilateral horn to support a pregnancy in the embryonic stage not the fetal stage (Sharma et al., 2010).

It is possible that young mares that did conceive on foal heat had better reproductive competence and, therefore, most likely to recover quickly from their previous pregnancy (Blanchard et al., 2004). In such mares, the ipsilateral horn is capable of supporting an embryo. Sharma et al., (2010) clearly identified that in lactating mares there is a higher risk of embryonic and overall pregnancy loss in pregnancies located in the uterine horn ipsilateral to the horn from which the mare delivered her most recent foal and is a point of further concern as it contributes substantially to the subfertility in the Thoroughbred mare population.

4.1.4. The Effect of Maternal Health and Body Condition on the Endocrine Responses of Neonatal Foals

Epidemiological observations in man have shown that the risk of adult onset degenerative diseases, such as hypertension and Type 2 diabetes, correlates with birth weight, independently of current weight or lifestyle in populations of different ages, gender and ethnic origin. Because intrauterine growth is determined primarily by the nutrient supply, the associations between birth weight and adult disease have been linked to por nutrition during early life. This has led to the concept that tissues are programmed in utero during critical periods of development by the availability of nutrients. Prenatal nutritional programming has been examined experimentally in a number of species using a range of techniques to manipulate the fetal nutrient supply. These studies all support the concept and have shown that nutrition during fetal life affects cardiovascular, metabolic and endocrine function in the mature individual. In particular, maternal undernutrition during either the whole of pregnancy or for discrete periods of gestation has been shown to affect adversely glucose tolerance, pancreatic endocrine function and insulin sensitivity in the mature offspring of rats, guinea pigs and sheep (Reusens and Remacle, 2006).

However, little is known about the postnatal consequences of nutritional manipulations during pregnancy in the horse. The horse is a precocious species the fetus of which matures relatively late in gestation; consequently it is more prone to prematurity and organ dysfunction than other experimental animals. Thoroughbred fillies, retired to stud as brood mares, are fed high energy rations, which are usually high in hydrolysable carbohydrate (sugar and starch) content, throughout pregnancy in an attempt to maximise fetal growth. In pubertal sheep, however, high energy intake during pregnancy tends to restrict rather than enhance placental and fetal growth. Similarly, feeding high fat diets to pregnant rats reduces birth weight and leads to insulin resistance in their adult offspring. Previous studies in the horse have shown that increasing the fetal nutrient supply by transferring small pony embryos into larger TB recipient mares increased placental and fetal growth and enhanced pancreaticβ cell function in the newborn foal (Allen et al., 2002). In contrast, restricting the fetal nutrient supply by transferring Thoroughbred embryos into smaller Pony mares did not alter β cell sensitivity to glucose but increased basal cortisol concentrations in association with reduced birth weight compared to control thoroughbred foals (Ousey, 2004).

Hyperadrenocortical function is also seen in newborn foals that are small at birth. However, the effects of the maternal nutritional plane, particularly over-nutrition, on the foal remain unknown (Ousey et al., 2008). However, this aim was confounded by an outbreak of *Streptococcus equi* that infected all mares at the start of the second trimester and caused maternal pyrexia, inappetence and weight loss. The final study, therefore investigated the neonatal consequences of an acute period of nutrient restriction superimposed upon different planes of nutrition, a scenario common in wild and domesticated equine populations.

4.1.5. Effect of Nutrition, Stress, Age and Environmental Factors on Embryonic and Placental Development

The equine placenta is nondeciduous, noninvasive, epitheliochorial and diffuse. From day 40 after ovulation, the allantochorion establishes a microvillous attachment to the lumenal epithelium of the endometrium and blunt villi interdigitate with from the surface of the endometrium. As gestation advances, continued branching of the villi leads to the formation of the mature microplacentome which maximises the surface area contact between maternal and fetal epithelial layers (Leiser et al., 1998).

Microplacentome development is essentially complete by 150 days gestation, although further remodelling of each structure continues until term (Abd-Elnaeim et al., 2006). Both age and parity have profound effects on the development of the microcotyledons on the surface of the Thoroughbred placenta, specifically. A reduction in the surface area, or plexiform nature, of the microcotyledons occurs in older mares suffering age-related degenerative changes (endometrosis) in the opposing endometrium, and also in young, primigravid mares (Wilsher and Allen, 2003). These events results in lower birthweight foals from both maiden and aged mares, compared with young and middle-aged multiparous mares. Surprisingly, however, assessment of placental efficiency in terms of kg foal birthweight/m^2 microscopic fetomaternal contact shows that the allantochorion of both primiparous and aged multiparous mares is more 'productive' than that of other groups of multiparous mares. Indeed, regardless of mare age and parity, microscopic surface area of the allantochorion is correlated negatively with placental efficiency.

Similar correlations matching increases in placental weight with decreases in efficiency have been reported in the pig, in which placental efficiency is also correlated positively with placental and endometrial vascularity (Wilson and Ford, 2001). To date, the differences observed in placental efficiency in the horse have not been related to placental vascularity, although changes in endometrial vascularity and maternal blood flow have been observed in mares of varying age and parity (Bollwein et al., 1999).

It is clear from work in other species that placental development can be enhanced or compromised by a variety of factors. In the ewe, for example, a critical period of sensitivity occurs between days 40 and 80 of gestation, which coincides with rapid proliferative growth of the placenta. During this period, placental growth may be modulated nutritionally by the size, body condition and degree of maturity of the ewe. Short-term nutritional insults can suppress placental and fetal growth in the ewe, which may result in long-term changes in physiology and metabolism of the offspring (McMullen et al., 2005). On the other hand, the combination of immaturity and over-nutrition might cause reductions in microcotyledon surface density and foal birthweight observed in primigravid vs. young multiparous mares (Wilsher and Allen, 2003).

4.1.5.1. The Effect of Age on Multiple Ovulation Rates, Multiple Pregnancy Rates and Embryonic Vesicle Diameter in the Mare

Reproductive competence, manifest as the production of a viable foal, is of paramount importance in equine stud management and, is therefore, of significant interest to breeders and veterinarians. Numerous factors have been reported to affect reproductive performance though many reports are conflicting. Further understanding of these factors should help to identify mares at greatest risk of pregnancy failure and so allow them to be carefully monitored. The age of the mare is reported by some to be one of these factors. Increasing age is known to be associated with poorer reproductive competence especially in mares 20 years of age or older (Carnevale et al., 2000).

This is manifest as lower pregnancy rates and increasing embryo mortality (Morris and Allen, 2002). Embryo mortality figures of 62% to 73% have been reported in mares over 15 years. The cause of such high embryo mortality rates is reported to include susceptibility to infection (Newcombe, 2000). Additionally the incidence of chronic endometrial disease (CED) is correlated to age and possibly parity, with the additional complication of reduced uterine tone and contractility (Carnevale and Ginther, 1992). Ovarian function is also reported to decline with age, ovarian weight, number of developing follicles and morphological normality of oocytes also suffering with age (Carnevale et al., 2000).

Other factors leading to depressed reproductive function in older mares include the increased incidence of multiple uterine cysts, and increased incidence of delayed involution (Newcombe, 2000). Increasing age may also have an effect on reproductive function more indirectly by an association with an increasing incidence of multiple ovulation (MO) (Davies Morel and O'Sullivan, 2001) and hence with increasing multiple pregnancies (MP). The mare, as a monocotous species, is very rarely able to successfully support MP to term. Evidence indicating an association between age and MO is conflicting, though some workers report a significant increase in MO with age, 15% of cycles yielding MO in 3 to 5-year olds compared with 35.1% of cycles in 18 to 22-year olds, 14% in 2 to 5-year olds compared with 18% in 6 to 10-year olds and 13% in 3 to 13-year olds compared with 24% in mares over 18 years of age. MP are correlated with MO, so it might also be expected that increasing age is associated with increasing MP. However, as already noted, increasing age is associated with increasing embryo mortality, possibly counteracting any affect of an increase in MO (Morris and Allen, 2002).

Finally, an effect of age on vesicle size may be an additional indirect effect on reproductive competence. Reports on the effect of vesicle size are again very limited. One report by Ball (1993) suggests that prior to day 2 there is no age effect. However, it is known that small for age vesicles are the ones most likely to fail, 62% to 78% vesicles identified as small at Days 12–14 were reported to subsequently fail (Ginther, 1986). It is hypothesized, (Davies Morel et al., 2005) that one of the reasons for high embryo mortality rates in older mares maybe an association between advancing age and small vesicle size.

4.1.5.2. Reproductive Efficiency of Intensively Managed Thoroughbred Mares

The Thoroughbred horse is considered to have relatively poor reproductive efficiency compared with sheep and beef cattle, selected for fertility, with target/cycle pregnancy rates >79% and live birth rates exceeding 90%. Pregnancy rates >85% for mares running with a stallion for 2 oestrous cycles have been reported and fertilisation rates of 90% (young, healthy) and 81% (older, subfertile) mares when oviducts were flushed 2–4 days postovulation (Ball, 1988). Retrospective studies of Thoroughbred, Standardbred and Quarter Horse mares revealed per cycle pregnancy rates of only 43–56%, cumulative end-of-season pregnancy rates of 70–80% (Brück et al.,, 1993) and foaling rates of 50–70% (Morley and Townsend, 1997).

Sanderson and Allen (1987) recorded that 1367 Thoroughbred mares mated in the Newmarket area, UK, during 1982, had an overall pregnancy rate/mated oestrous cycle of 52.4%, a rate of 88.7% at examination 60–90 days after the last mating and a live foal birth rate the following year of 74.7%. Analysis of Weatherby's Stud Book records for 12.386 mares mated in the same year (1982) revealed that 80.5% ended the season pregnant and 71.4% foaled. This suggests that pregnancy failure contributes substantially to the relatively low levels of reproductive efficiency encountered in the Thoroughbred. Thoroughbred mares and stallions are selected, not on fertility traits, but almost entirely upon a combination of pedigree and performance on the racetrack; and physiological and managerial factors may contribute to the failure of mares to conceive and/or carry a pregnancy to term. The mare is a long day seasonal breeder and there is a disparity between their physiological mating season (april to october in the northern hemisphere) and that arbitrarily imposed for the purposes of agerelated racing (mid-february to early july), and many mares are hand-mated to individual stallions within a 4 month period (february to july). Age and status of the mare as maiden, barren or lactating also influence the chances of conceiving and producing a live foal. These various mare factors, together with the management of the stallion contribute greatly to the overall reproductive efficiency of any group of horses (Sanderson and Allen, 1987).

4.1.5.3. Effects of Exercise or Oocyte Heat Shock on Embryo Development and Gene Expression in the Horse

Efficiency of reproduction is of vital importance to the equine industry. Many complex processes are involved in reproduction and interruption during any of these steps can lead to failure of the mare to conceive or maintain pregnancy. Many owners today maintain their mares in competition and/or training throughout the breeding season. These owners utilize the reproductive technology of embryo transfer to allow their mares to remain in training while being bred and may unwittingly be lessening their chances of recovering an embryo. If an embryo is recovered, it may be of poorer quality and/or retarded in its growth, thus reducing their chances for a foal. In comparison with other species of livestock, horses are often seen as inefficient in conception and maintenance of pregnancy. This in reality is a misconception. Due to the demands we have placed on the horse, particularly the annual January 1st birth date for most breed registries, producers try to breed their horses early in the calendar year, outside of their natural breeding season. Other factors that may induce stress such as transport and/or heat have the capacity to suppress conception rates (Squires et al., 2003).

It is common for young, valuable mares to remain in training throughout the breeding season, with the owner utilizing embryo transfer to prevent interruption of the mare's training and/or competition schedule (Squires et al., 2003). Exercise or training can possibly alter the reproductive cycle of mares and/or lessen their chance to conceive a viable embryo. One of the byproducts of exercise is a substantial increase of heat in the horse. Exercise for as little as 30 minutes can lead to a body temperature increase of 2.5 ºC (McCutcheon and Geor, 2000). Exercise also stimulates a stress hormonal response, and an increase in corticosteroids has been shown to suppress important reproductive hormones such as GnRH and LH (Kalantaridou, et al., 2004). Sertich (1989) reported a depressed rate of 40.5 % in embryos recovered in performance mares over a 4 years period. All of the mares studied were maintained in training and competition during the breeding season.

This is in contrast to reported embryo recovery rates of a slightly higher 50% (Squires et al., 2003) and up to an optimal 75% rate (Vogelsang et al., 1985). The lower recovery reported by Sertich (1989) may be due to individual mare or stallion fertility, or to recovery technique, as no control mares were utilized in that report. However it is possible a slightly lower embryo recovery rate is found in performance mares. Supporting this, among the veterinary community, it is often perceived that mares subjected to work have inferior fertility rates; mares that remain in competition during the breeding season produce fewer embryos and/or fail to conceive (Mortensen, 2007).

4.1.5.4. Heat Stress Reproductive Performance

Hansen et al.,(2001) states that it is likely that reproductive function will be compromised in a cow whose body temperature increases approximately 1°C or more for a period of more than 4 hours, indicating that temperatures above homeothermy can disrupt maternal reproductive function. The reproductive processes in the male and female mammal are very sensitive to disruption by hyperthermia with the most pronounced consequences being reduced quantity and quality of sperm production in males and decreased oocyte and early embryonic developmental competence in females.

In mares, the heat stress associated with exercising also is related with alterations of dynamics of estrous cycle. The mares exercised ovulates significantly smaller follicles than they did when not under exercise, and this may be an indication of impaired folliculogenesis. Furthermore, mares exercised have significant delays in time to ovulation after luteolysis with PGF2α, indicating that the exercise affect timing of ovulation with possible impairment of folliculogenesis. The ovulation of smaller follicles seen in these mares is similar to what has been observed in cattle. Wilson et al., (1998) reported that heat stressed heifers had smaller dominant second wave follicles. Consequentially, the heifers in their study had a longer estrous cycle. Rensis and Scaramuzzi (2003) reported that heat stress in cow delays follicle selection and lengthen the follicular wave, thus interrupting and lengthening the estrous cycle. How these two abnormalities in the estrous cycle affect mare fertility is not clear, however, Hansen et al., (2001) stated that disruption in patterns of folliculogenesis, leading to a lengthened period of dominance for the largest follicle, leads to poor fertility. Mihm et al., (1999) reported that in cattle with lengthened follicular dominance (>9 day), oocytes ovulated had reduced competence. These trends observed in cattle could possibly be associated with the poorer fertility seen in the mares on the decreased embryo recovery rate.

Heat stress has been associated with poor conception rates in many species. This may not only be due to poor oocyte quality but also to disruption of the process of fertilization and/or early embryonic development. Increased average daily heat and humidity above 21°C on a day prior to breeding it is associated with a significant linear decrease in conception rates in dairy cattle (Ingraham et al., 1974). Indeed, this latter authors reported conception rates for cows serviced with an average heat index under 18.9 °C was 67%, compared to cows serviced on day averaging above 24.4 °C was 21%. Besides, Lenz et al., (1983) stated that the production of hyaluronic acid by the cumuli, occurrence of the acrosome reaction in sperm cells, and fertilization are all temperature-dependent processes and under elevated temperatures may be disrupted, causing reproductive failure.

Poor reproductive performance associated with thermal stress may be due to high temperature acting directly on the developing embryo with early embryonic development possibly compromised by heat stress (Putney et al., 1989; Rivera and Hansen, 2001). During the early cleavage stages of embryonic development, the embryonic genome is largely suppressed (Al-Katani and Hansen, 2002) and the developing embryo is dependent upon the proteins and RNA stored by the oocyte for survival and further development. The equine genome is not thought to be active until the 4-8 cells stage and early equine embryonic development is comparable to other species.

Temperatures that have little effect on survival of most cells can be lethal to preimplantation embryos (Rivera et al., 2003). Putney et al., (1989) stated that the early bovine embryo is extremely sensitive to maternal heat stress prior to day 7 of embryonic development, which may severely compromise its viability and may lead to an increased rate of early embryonic mortality. The detrimental effect of heat stress on early embryonic development may be multi-factorial, with effects seen on the intrauterine environment and/or direct effects on the conceptus.

The intrauterine environment is compromised in heat-stressed cows with a decrease in blood flow to the uterus and increased uterine temperature. These changes can inhibit embryonic development, increase early embryonic loss and reduce the proportion of successful inseminations (Rensis and Scaramuzzi, 2003). In contrast, Wettemann and Bazer (1985) reported that heat stress does not appear to alter uterine blood flow in gilts, although fertility is reduced.

Elevated uterine temperature may result in an increase in the metabolic rate of the bovine conceptus and thus, alter nutrient uptake and growth. Increased conceptus metabolic rate, as well as decreases in nutrient secretion by the uterus, may result in retarded development. In agreement with this concept, Putney et al., (1989) stated that high environmental temperature may severely alter bovine conceptus metabolic activity in vivo and lead to reduced growth rates and failure of the conceptus to produce biochemical signals in adequate amounts for pregnancy recognition and maintenance of CL function. Furthermore, high oviductal and uterine temperatures may have directly altered the metabolic activity of stressed embryos, resulting in developmental retardation and a reduced rate of embryonic growth. Also, Ryan et al., (1992) reported in cattle that chronic elevation of temperature above the normal culture temperature (40 vs. 38.6 ºC) in vitro resulted in a higher incidence of embryo death that was evident shortly after embryo hatching. Biggers et al., (1987) reported pregnancy rates and day 17 conceptus wet weights were significantly lower in heat-stressed groups and these embryos were less than half the weight of embryos from non-heat stressed cows.

During early embryonic cleavage, the majority of the embryo cell cycle is spent in the synthesis (S) and mitotic (M) phases.The S and M phases are disrupted by elevated temperatures; exposure of cells to heat shock during the S phase results in spontaneous premature chromosome condensation and micronuclear formation while heat shock during the M phase results in disassembly of the mitotic spindle, failure of cytokinesis and polyploidy (Swanson et al., 1995). Rivera et al., (2003) reported that disruption of development caused by exposure of two-cell bovine embryos to a physiologically relevant heat shock (41ºC-6 h) involves alterations to the cytoskeleton and mitochondria. Elevated temperatures in vitro caused alterations in the nucleus, cytoplasm, mitochondria, and other organelles of early embryonic cells. Some of the changes, particularly to the cytoskeleton and mitochondria, occur at temperatures characteristic of cows experiencing hyperthermia-induced infertility. When mitochondria are damaged they can no longer maintain a proton gradient, aerobic ATP synthesis is arrested, a progressive unfolding of the inner mitochondrial cristae occurs, and several apoptosis initiator components such as cytochrome c and apoptosis-inducing factor are released. In addition, heat shock damages the nucleus, induces protein aggregation and functional and ultrastructural changes in membranes. These results reported in bovine embryos are in agreement with the report of Coss and Linnemans (1996) in which heat shock induced morphological alterations to the cytoskeleton in hamster embryos and hindered further development.

On the contrary, embryos become more resistant to heat stress as pregnancy progresses (Hansen et al., 2001). Ealy et al., (1994) observed that embryos were sensitive to deleterious effects of maternal heat stress at day 1 of pregnancy but became more resistant to heat stress effects by day 3. These authors suggested that increased embryonic heat tolerance in day 3 and older bovine embryos may be due to the ability of the embryos to produce heat-shock proteins after activation of the embryonic genome at the 8-to 16-cells stage. Latter, Rivera et al., (2003) found that hypersensitivity of the pre-implantation embryo to elevated temperatures is a transient phenomenon; effects of heat shock on the development of cultured bovine embryos were reduced as embryos advanced in development past the 2 to 4-cells stage.

4.1.5.5. The Effect of Exercise on Folliculogenesis, Cortisol, Estradiol and Luteinizing Hormone in Mares

Many horse owners utilize artificial reproductive technologies to allow their mares to remain in training and produce offspring (Squires et al., 2003). It has been perceived that mares in competition during the breeding season produce fewer embryos and/or fail to conceive. There is little information on the effects of heat stress or exercise on mare reproductive efficiency. Sertich (1989) reported an embryo recovery rate of 40.5% in 111 uterine flushes of performance mares in training and competition over a 4-year period. Typical embryo recovery rates of non-exercised mares range between 50 to 75%. Mortensen et al., (2009) reported mares exercised daily for 30 min under hot and humid conditions achieved rectal temperature increases from 38.0°C to 39.9°C and had a significantly reduced embryo recovery rate than non-exercised mares, 63% versus 34%, respectively. Additionally, these researchers reported ovulations from smaller follicles and an increased time from PGF2α administration to subsequent ovulation in exercised mares compared with control mares. Stress has been shown to reduce fertility in livestock animals. Stress is described as the inability of an animal to cope with its environment, a disruption of homeostasis; an induction of allostasis, or the state of an organism under the influence of external or internal forces which alter its dynamic equilibrium (Mastorakos et al., 2005). Exercise is a physical stressor that challenges homeostasis and affects five major categories of biological function: 1) stress responses, 2) availability and utilization of metabolic energy, 3) maintenance of homeostasis, 4) growth and maintenance of cardiac and skeletal muscle, and 5) reproduction.

The stress response can be mediated by the nervous system and/or by hormones produced by the endocrine system. Several hormones of importance for reproduction and maintenance of homeostasis during and after exercise are produced by the anterior and posterior lobes of the pituitary gland. The hypothalamus acts as an integrator in the controlled system, exerting control over the pituitary through neural and endocrine mechanisms. During exercise, the adrenal glands increase production of epinephrine, norepinephrine and corticosteroids (McKeever, 2002).

There have been several studies examining the effect of exercise on various stress and metabolic hormones; as well as several studies examining the effect of stress on reproduction. In horses, there are limited data on the impact of exercise on folliculogenesis. Evidence suggests that mares in training experienced decreased fertility when measured by embryo recovery rate (Mortensen et al., 2009). Both studies reported a decrease in embryo recovery rates in exercised mares. Additional information suggests that exercise may have an effect on folliculogenesis in mares as shown by decreased diameter of the ovulatory follicle at the time of ovulation.

There is increasing evidence of exercise related short-term and long-term consequences in female athlete that many authors described as "exercise-related female reproductive dysfunction" (Mastorakos et al., 2005). The Hypothalamic Pituitary Gonadal axis (HPG) exerts an inhibitory effect on the female reproductive system.

Reproduction could be potentially inhibited by components of the stress pathways and activation of stress systems that potentially influence reproduction at any level of the HPG axis. Corticotropin-releasing factor (CRF) inhibits GnRH secretion, while glucocorticoids suppress LH, ovarian estrogen and P_4 secretion; consequentially, rendering target tissues resistant to estradiol. While it is possible stress may directly influence the gonads, it is generally accepted that the predominant influence is on the secretion of GnRH, LH, and FSH (Kalantaridou et al., 2004).

The female reproductive system is highly sensitive to physiological stress, and reproductive abnormalities including delayed menarche, primary and secondary amenorrhea and oligomenorrhea. Menstrual abnormalities in the female athlete result from suppression of the spontaneous pulsatile hypothalamic secretion of GnRH, which results in decreased pulsatile secretion of LH and FSH and shuts down stimulation of the ovary. A number of factors, such as energy balance, exercise intensity, training practices, bodyweight, fat composition, eating disorders, and physical and emotional stress may contribute to the development of female athletic dysfunction. The stress of exercise, the concomitant activation of the HPG axis, and the observed hypercortisolemia are some of the main factors that lead to suppression of the HPG axis (Mastorakos et al., 2005). Increases in glucocorticoids may be causally linked to the inhibition of reproductive function that is another physiological correlation that often accompanies stress (Daley et al., 2000).

Administration of natural or synthetic glucocorticoids has an anti-gonadal effect in rodents, horses, primates and sheep. Asa and Ginther (1982) reported mares treated with dexamethasone, a synthetic glucocorticoid, only 1 of 8 mares exhibited estrous behavior and only 2 appeared to ovulate. This suggested a negative feedback action of dexamethasone on the pituitary or hypothalamic mechanisms controlling release of LH. The ability of dexamethasone to interfere with ovulation suggested a potential influence of adrenal gland secretions on the reproductive physiology of the mare. Furthemore, transport as origin of stress in mares (Baucus et al., 1990).

Research results suggested that cortisol may act indirectly via the hypothalamus to elicit a mediator that acts on the pituitary to inhibit response to GnRH in diverse species (Brandt et al., 2009). It is possible that undisturbed communication with the hypothalamus is required to maintain cells in the pituitary responsive to regulatory molecules, such as cortisol. Elevated plasma cortisol concentrations are correlated with signs of stress in mammals.

One potential complication of studying the effect of stress on reproduction is that the varying endocrine status throughout the estrous cycle may modulate the response to stress. Indeed, estradiol infused intravenously at a rate of 65.6 ng/kg/hr in Rhesus monkey appeared to enhance the inhibitory effect of glucocorticoids on gonadotropin secretion.

In rodents, there is evidence that sex steroids may interact with both the central and peripheral substrates of stress, possibly modifying the HPG axis response. Indeed, the negative feedback of estradiol results in reduced activity of the hypothalamic GnRH pulse generating system and decreased gonadotropin secretion. It is interesting to note that this response to stress is particularly acute during the follicular phase of the reproductive cycle and less prominent in ovariectomized animals or animals in the luteal phase (Daley et al., 2000).

4.1.5.6. Foaling Rates and Risk Factors for Abortion in Pregnant Mares in Relation to Colic

Colic is one of the most difficult diseases to study with epidemiologic methods due to the large number of diseases, which create the signs of colic. Making a specific diagnosis is not always possible in horses with colic; therefore classification of the simple colic is a challenge (White, 2005). Information about incidence, mortality, and risk factors is helpful to the clinician in making decisions about individual cases as well as herd problems.

Colic is responsible for more deaths in horses that any disease group except for old age.

In the normal farm population, horse mortality from all types of colic was 0.7 deaths per 100 horse-year with a colic case fatality rate of 6.7%. In one study case fatalities were due to stomach rupture, strangulating lesions or enteritis (Tinker, 1995).

Determining the cause of different diseases that cause colic is problematic since only natural disease has been studied. In some cases the cause may be evident such as in the case of grain overload, or an enterolith but even in these cases the mechanism which initiates the problem is often unknown. By determining risk factor the cause may be elaborated, and it is often possible to reduce the incidence of colic be decreasing exposure to the incriminated risk. The amount of risk is stated as the odds that the colic incidence will increase in a group of horses exposed to a particular factor compared to the colic incidence in a group that is not exposed to that factor. Observations in several studies have suggested that Arabian horses have more colic when other studies have reported more colic in Thoroughbreds. Standardbred, gaited horse and Warmblood stallions appear to have more inguinal hernias due to the increased size of their inguinal rings. Though rare, the recessive and lethal trait of aganglionosis occurs in paint foals born to overo mares mated with overo stallions and so far the only genetically linked disease recognized to cause colic (White, 2005).

Horses having a history of colic were at higher risk for more colic episodes (Tinker et al., 1997). Also, horses, which had previous abdominal surgery, were also at higher risk of repeat colic which in most cases is felt to be due to adhesions or bowel scarring with stricture. Parasites have been related to an increased colic risk by several studies. Obstructions due to ascarids, strongyle infection has been related to increase colic and specifically with colic associated with diseases of ileum and cecum including increasing the rate of ileocecal intussusception and cecocecal intussusception (Proudman and Holdstock, 2000).

Horse transport increased the risk of colic risk. This has been suspected by practitioners, who commonly administer a laxative prior to shipping to prevent colic from impactions. The mechanism or cause of the increased incidence is unknown. When combining risks of transport, feeding grain and cribbing the risk were markedly increased (Tinker, 1995).

Veterinarians and owners frequently associate weather changes with increased frequency of colic, but most of the previous studies have been unable to find statistical proof of increased risk.

Cold weather which affects water intake has been linked to increased impaction colic. Most likely the focal increase in colic episodes was not directly related to the weather, but rather due to management changes caused by the weather. Horses consuming hard water, alfalfa hay and with a higher pH and mineral concentrations of colon ingesta, are at higher risk for this problem (White, 2005).

Pregnant mares that are presened with colic requiring medical or surgical treatment may be at risk of fetal loss due to untoward effects of illness, anesthesia, and surgery on fetal viability. For example, horses with colic may have varying degrees of systemic illness, including severe dehydration and signs of endotoxemia. In the pregnant mare, these conditions may put the fetus at great risk. Previous studies have suggested that pretreatment with flunixin meglumine reduces the risk of abortion in mares suffering endotoxemia by preventing PF2α release by the endometrium and resultant lysis of the CL (Daels et al., 1991). Pregnant mares suffering colic are commonly administered P_4, with the assumption that it will reduce the risk of abortion due to the mare's illness (Macpherson, 2006).

The mare has been reported to have a higher risk for colon displacement or volvulus during late pregnancy or lactation. However, all studies have been based on selected populations of mares or in regions with high numbers of broodmares. When compared for exposure for events in a Virginia-Maryland Study, mares had an increased risk of colic from 60 to 150 days after foaling (Proudman, 1992). The physiologic events which predispose to this increased risk are not known, but calcium levels and alterations in diet including increases in energy due to more concentrates in the diet to support lactation may be related to this increased risk.

The risk of postoperative abortion in mares undergoing surgery for colic is surprisingly low, and not related to stage of gestation or type of lesion. In a retrospective study, Santschi et al., (1991a,b) found that 18% of surviving mares that underwent colic surgery experienced pregnancy loss. Half of the abortions occurred long after the resolution of the disease, and may have been unrelated to the surgery or colic. Hypoxia and endotoxemia were identified as risk factors associated with death of the fetus. Abortions were associated with a PO2 <80 mm Hg when surgery occurred during the last two months of gestation.

Uterine torsion usually presents as a mild colic during the last trimester of pregnancy. Diagnosis is based primarily on rectal palpation of the broad ligaments. When the uterus is torsed, the mare is at risk for uterine rupture. Options for correction include rolling the mare, or surgical correction. Rolling may be an alternative to surgery early in the third trimester, but should not be tried in mares close to term due to increased risk of uterine rupture. Surgical correction is the most effective treatment for uterine torsion, and was found to result in the highest survival rate of foals. Furthermore, the prognosis for mares and foals is best when uterine torsion occurs at <320 days of gestation (Chaney et al., 2006).

5. Infectious Causes of Embryonic and Fetal Mortality

Although more deaths occur at and around birth than between 1 week of age and weaning, embryonic losses are usually higher than perinatal losses. Notably, maternal infections during pregnancy may or may not impact fetal development.

The impact on fetal development may be caused directly by infectious agents or their toxins, or indirectly by placentitis. Furthermore, detection of a reproductive pathogen should not preclude further diagnostic testing, as dual infections are not uncommon. Embryonic or fetal death may result in resorption, mummification, maceration, or abortion. Aborted fetuses may be autolytic due to death 24–48 hours before abortion. Fetal mummification occurs most commonly in polytocous species (e.g. swine). Bacterial infections are usually not involved in mummification; however, viruses are a common cause of mummification in pigs, dogs, and cats. Fetal maceration results when abortion or parturition fails to occur following fetal death and CL regression (Givens and Marley, 2008).

Pathogens that cause sporadic reproductive loss in mares may be due primarily to host factors, e.g. impaired reproductive defense mechanisms. Notably, other pathogens may cause disease, depending on variables of the environment (e.g. movement of horses that predisposes mares to novel infections). *Streptococcus zooepidemicus (S. zooepidemicus)* is one of the most common bacteria isolated from mares with uterine disease. Whereas the uterus of a healthy mare is more likely to clear the infection, the uterus of a mare with impaired defense mechanisms or poor genital conformation might become inflamed or develop an infection leading to infertility. As well, *S. zooepidemicus* can cause abortion via ascension through the cervix and infection of the fetus and placenta, or possibly through a maternal systemic infection. Bacterial abortions usually occur at 5 to 10 months of gestation. In addition to bacterial culture, diagnosis of infection is coupled with evidence of autolysis and inflammation of the fetus and placenta. Other bacteria implicated in infertility or abortion are *E. coli, Pseudomonas aeruginosa, Klebsiella pneumoniae var genitalium, Staphylococcus aureus, Streptococcus equisimilis, Leptospira spp., S. abortus equi,* and nocardioform actinomycetes. Although no longer very common, *S. abortus equi* has caused abortion outbreak in one of these, 21 of 26 mares aborted between 5 and 10 months of gestation (Madic et al., 1997).

Taylorella equigenitalis is a gram-negative coccobacillus that causes contagious equine metritis (CEM). *T. equigenitalis* is transmitted venereally, highly contagious, and can cause a copious vulvar discharge. Diagnosis is by bacteriologic culture of the organism from the clitoral fossa, clitoral sinuses, and endometrium or cervix. As well, polymerase chain reaction can be used to identify the organism. Serologic tests are also available to detect antibodies against Taylorella equigenitalis in the serum. Most mares recover spontaneously from CEM over a period of several months. Imported horses used for breeding should be quarantined and extensively tested. Any animals suspected of having CEM should be reported to state or federal animal health authorities (Givens and Marley, 2008).

Equine herpesvirus 1 (EHV-1) can cause abortion, neonatal death, respiratory disease, and neurologic disease. The virus is transmitted through inhalation of infectious aerosol droplets, or by direct contact with infectious secretions. Like other herspesviruses, equine herpesvirus 1 persists in a latent state that can be reactivated. Most abortions are sporadic and occur between 7 months of gestation and term. The abortions can occur up to 4 months after respiratory disease, which may have been clinical, or subclinical (Swerczek and Dennis, 2007a).

Equine viral arteritis can cause sporadic abortions between 5 and 10 months of gestation (Swerczek and Dennis, 2007b). The virus is transmitted by inhalation of infectious aerosol droplets or venereally. If clinical signs of disease are apparent, they can consist of fever, hind limb edema, nasal and ocular discharge, urticarial rash, anorexia, coughing, and dyspnea. The virus can also cause uterine disease, with subsequent abortion in pregnant mares (Coignoul and Cheville, 1984).

Trypanosoma equiperidum is a venereally transmitted protozoa that causes dourine. Although it has been eradicated from North America and most of Europe, the disease is still found in Africa, South and Central America, and the Middle East. Clinical signs include a mucopurulent vulvar discharge, fever, and cutaneous raised plaques followed by ataxia, depression, severe anemia, and death. Mortality can reach 50–70%. Strict quarantine, testing, and eradication of positive animals are recommended for control of the disease (Samper and Tibary, 2006).

Fungal pathogens account for up to 10% of reported sporadic abortions (Swerczek and Dennis, 2007c). *Aspergillus fumigatus* is the most common fungal pathogen, but *Mucor spp* and *Allescheria boydii* have also been reported. Infection of the uterus may occur via ascension through the cervix or hematogenously. Abortions usually occur at 8 to 11 months of gestation, and may be associated with a purulent vulvar discharge. The affected chorioallantois is thickened, yellowish, and covered with a mucoid exudate.

5.1. Levels of Selected T Lymphocyte Subpopulations in Peripheral Blood of Mares Which Experienced Embryonic Death

Early embryonic death (EED) in mares is defined as gestation failure within 40 days after insemination. Embryos die at various stages of their development, starting from fertilized eggs, through morules, blastocysts to older embryos undergoing organogénesis. Hence, two periods of EED are distinguished. The first period is from fertilization to post-ovulation day 11. The second period is from days 14 to 40 when the embryo is already in the uterus. According to many authors, EED is most commonly caused by infectious endometritis (Portus et al., 2005). This inflammation may develop within the first few hours following mating or artificial insemination (Troedsson et al., 2001). The inflammation results from reactions of local protective mechanisms to the semen and its impurities containing non-specific bacterial flora. The response to an antigen results in the influx of neutrophils into the uterine lumen leading to phagocytosis. During this process, PGF2α is released, which increases myometrial contractility and promotes the clearance of the remaining semen and bacteria (Portus et al., 2005). With efficient cell defence mechanisms and normal myometrial contractility the inflammation is quickly cleared from the uterus within 36–48 h (Troedsson et al., 2001).

Impaired uterine clearance of inflammatory products due to dysfunction of local defence mechanisms results in chronic endometritis, increased concentrations of PGF2α, luteolysis of the CL and embryo loss (Troedsson, 2007). The literature data demonstrate that after the genome activation, the embryo synthesizes numerous proinflammatory cytokines and growth factors.

This is to provide suitable uterine conditions for implantation and further development of the embryo (Betancourt-Alonso et al., 2006).

Normal pregnancy is accompanied by the immune inflammatory response, which is mainly induced and modulated by cytokines of pro- and anti-inflammatory action (Daher et al., 2004). Furthemor, in early pregnancy, T lymphocytes are activated by fetal antigens (Piccinni et al., 2000). Studies have demonstrated that in pregnant females the CD4+/CD8+ ratio disproportion led to early or late embryonic death (Wattegedera et al., 2008). This is due to proinflammatory cytokines produced by Th1 lymphocytes (IL1, IL2 and IL6 etc., which activate NK cells responsible for cytolytic effects of trophoblast cells and pregnancy losses (Krakowski et al., 2010).

5.2. Endometritis and Placentitis

5.2.1. Ascending Placentitis in the Mare

Placentitis in mares poses a significant threat to fetal and neonatal viability. Placentitis is commonly caused by bacteria ascending through the vagina. The most frequent bacterial pathogens implicated in equine placentitis are *Streptococcus equi* subspecies *zooepidemicus*, *Escherichia coli*, *Klebsiella pneumonia*, and *Pseudomonas aeruginosa*. While bacterial infection initiates disease, recent work from an experimental model of ascending placentitis in pony mares showed that premature delivery may occur secondary to inflammation of the chorion rather than as a consequence of fetal infection (Mays et al., 2002). It was suggested that these inflammatory processes may result in prostaglandin production (PGE_2 and PGF2α) and stimulation of myometrial contractility, thus resulting in preterm delivery.

However, in some chronic cases of placentitis, foals will experience accelerated fetal maturation. These foals will be delivered prematurely, but will be mature enough to survive in the extrauterine environment. In humans, it is thought that indirect stimulation of the fetal HPG axis by pro-inflammatory cytokines is responsible for precocious fetal maturation (Gravett et al., 2000). If this phenomenon is also true for equine fetuses, then delaying premature labor long enough to allow accelerated fetal maturation to occur may improve foal survival rates. To achieve this goal, it is necessary to promptly diagnose and effectively treat the disease. The most common signs of placentitis in mares are premature udder development and vulvar discharge.

Transrectal ultrasonographic examination of the caudal reproductive tract has become a commonplace diagnostic tool for placentitis. This method enables direct examination of the cervical star region, the area most often afflicted with placentitis. It also allows for evaluation of fetal activity, fetal fluid character, fetal orbit measures, and subjective amniotic evaluation. In the normal pregnant mare, the area visualized in the region of the cervical star is the combined uterine and placental (chorioallantoic) unit. Renaudin et al., (1999a) developed the technique for evaluation of the combined thickness of the uterus and placenta (CTUP) and established normal values in light-horse mares throughout gestation. For 271 to 300, 301 to 330, and >330 days of gestation, normal concentrations for CUTP were <8, <10, and <12 mm, respectively (Renaudin et al., 1999b). However, mares with placental infection or inflammation have increased (thicker) CTUP measures, or separation of the membranes from the endometrium. Furthermore, purulent material (hyperechoic) may accumulate in pockets between the chorioallantois and the endometrium. Thickening of the amnion may also indicate inflammation. Allantoic fluid throughout most of gestation is hypoechoic (black), whereas amniotic fluid is slightly more echodense (light gray). However, fetal activity can agitate cellular material and change the characteristics of either fluid compartment. Fluids that persistently have increased echodensity likely have increased cellularity due to infection or inflammation. Serial ultrasound examinations are essential to determine if fluid character changes are iatrogenic or pathologic (Macpherson and Bailey, 2008).

Transabdominal ultrasonography is an excellent tool for evaluating the fetus and placenta in mares. Placental membrane integrity and thickness and fetal fluid character are also evaluated using this technique. Again, the chorioallantois is intimately associated with the endometrium and cannot be easily identified as a separate structure from the transabdominal approach. Mares with normal pregnancies should have a minimum CTUP of 7.1±1.6 mm, and a maximal CTUP of 11.5±2.4 mm (Reef et al., 1996). Evaluation of the caudal allantochorion is not accurate using the transabdominal approach. However, transabdominal evaluation of fetal membranes is very useful for identifying placental abnormalities in mares with hematogenously-induced or nocardia-form placentitis. Mares infected with the nocardia-form bacteria will often have placental separation and purulent material at the base of the gravid horn and the junction of the uterine body (Hong et al., 1993).

Transrectal and transabdominal ultrasound, combined with endocrine-ological assays, provide additional tools for early diagnosing and monitoring progression of placentitis in mares. Unfortunately, many mares do not exhibit classical signs of infection, premature udder development and a vaginal discharge, so infections are commonly missed. Mares having vaginal discharge with or without udder development should be examined ultrasonographically (LeBlanc, 2010).

Ultrasonographic changes in the placental unit may be seen transrectally, especially in the cervical region, or transabdominally in cases of Nocardioform placentitis. Most placental lesions are observed by transrectal ultrasonography as over 90% of cases are caused by ascending infections. The combined thickness of the uterus and placenta (CTUP) should be measured in the ventral portion of the uterus, just cranial to the cervix. The CTUP increases from a mean of 4.0 mm between 4 and 8 months to 1.0 to 1.2 cm at term (Renaudin et al., 1997). A CTUP greater than 1.2 cm at 9 months of gestation or a CTUP greater than 1.5 cm at 11 months is associated with ascending placentitis. The fetal membranes may separate from the uterus, and pus may be visualized swirling between the membranes and uterus. Mares that exhibit premature udder development without a vaginal discharge should be evaluated by transabdominal ultrasonography for twins and Nocardioform placentitis. Uterine infections caused by Nocardioform organisms, an organism that resides in the soil, commonly result in abortion or premature delivery (LeBlanc, 2010).

Mares with placental pathology may have increased plasma concentrations of progestagens as a result of stress to the fetal placental unit (Rossdale et al.,, 1991). Fetal-placental P_4 is rapidly metabolized to 5α-pregnanes. Unfortunately, 5α-pregnanes are not readily assayed in a commercial setting, so diagnosis of placental disease using 5α-pregnane concentrations is not possible. This progestins cross-react with the P_4 antibody used in commercial radioimmunoassay and enzymelinked immunosorbent assays, and can be measured in the maternal circulation in late gestation (Ousey et al., 2005; Morris et al., 2007). Also, subnormal plasma relaxin concentrations were detected in mares with abnormal pregnancies. Mares with clinical signs of placentitis and mares exhibiting signs of fescue toxicosis had suppressed plasma relaxin concentrations. Furthermore, sensitivity assays can be improved when combined with evidence of placental thickening as detected using transrectal ultrasonography (Troedsson, 2007).

Premature delivery of a weak foal is devastating to horse owners, because most foals, if they live, never have productive performance careers even if they receive the best neonatal care. The single most important cause of premature delivery in the USA is placentitis. It accounts for nearly a third of late-term abortions and fetal mortality in the first day of life (Giles et al.,

1993). Placentitis affects approximately 3% to 7% of pregnant mares, the value of the foals, both economically and emotionally, makes this an important disease to study (LeBlanc, 2009).

Mares most commonly afflicted are pluriparous. Many have anatomical defects of the caudal reproductive tract such as pneumovagina, vestibule-vaginal reflux or cervical fibrosis, tears or adhesions. Some, but not all mares, exhibit a vaginal discharge and develop an udder prematurely in response to placentitis. Management of mares at risk of abortion owing to placentitis is directed at prolonging pregnancy because chronic placentitis has been associated with accelerated fetal maturation (Rossdale et al., 1992). A foal may be born significantly premature and survive with limited neonatal care, if premature birth can be delayed for a few weeks after placentitis develops (LeBlanc et al., 2004; Christiansen et al., 2009).

Treatment protocols designed for prolonging gestation and for producing viable foals are currently being studied in experimental models (Christiansen et al., 2009). Induction of parturition prematurely with the expectation of delivering a mature foal is not an option, because fetal maturation only occurs in the last 5 days of gestation and gestation length varies widely from 320 to 365 days. Removing the foetus from its dam's uterus before the narrow window of final maturation will result in a premature foal that will likely not survive even in the best of neonatal units. Inducing precocious maturation of the equine foetus with corticosteroids has been considered a risk and not reliable in mares at risk of premature birth. Due large doses are required (100 mg q 24 h for 3 days), data are limited and laminitis may be a séquela (Ousey et al., 2006).

Endometritis in the mare can be divided into acute infectious, chronic infectious or post–mating-induced endometritis. The most critical component in preventing the disease is rapid physical clearance of uterine contents after foaling and mating. Physical clearance can be hindered by anatomical abnormalities such as a pendulous uterus or incompetent cervix or by degenerative changes such as decreased uterine contractility, vascular elastosis or lymphangectasia. Mares with susceptibility to endometritis had one or more "risk factors".

Risk factors included abnormal reproductive history, abnormal perineal conformation, vulvoplasty not repaired after foaling, an incompetent cervix, positive endometrial culture, ≥2 cm of endometrial fluid before breeding, endometrial fluid post-mating between 1.5 and 2.0 cm, or a fluid volume ≥2 cm, and endometrial fluid persisting more than 36 hours after mating (LeBlanc, 2009; 2010).

Accumulation of uterine fluid during the ovulatory period is consistently associated with decreased pregnancy rates. The presence of two or more centimetres of intra-uterine fluid during oestrus or between 6 and 36 hours post-breeding are good indicators that a mare is susceptible to mating-induced endometritis (Brinsko et al., 2003; Bucca et al., 2008). In a recent study, intra-uterine fluid during oestrus was associated with increased numbers of neutrophils in the uterine lumen. Thoroughbred mares with intra-uterine fluid on day 2 or 3 of oestrus were 1.4 times more likely to have >5 neutrophils / 400x field on cytological specimens than those with no or mild inflammation (Burleson et al., 2010). However, intra-uterine fluid during oestrus was not always associated with bacterial endometritis.

Thoroughbred mares from which the bacterial organisms, *E. coli, Staphylococcus aureus, Pseudomonas spp.*, or bacteria considered to be non-pathogens (micro-coccus, alpha streptococcus or bacillus) were isolated had intra-uterine fluid in <40% of the ultrasonographic examinations (17–39% depending on organism) conducted immediately before the uterine culture was obtained. Intra-uterine fluid was seen more frequently, in 45–55% of the ultrasonographic examinations, when *Streptococcus b-haemolytic, Klebsiella pneumoniae, Enterobacter cloacae*, or yeast were isolated (Burleson et al., 2010). Other ultrasonographic abnormalities associated with decreased pregnancy rates include abnormal oedema patterns such as excessive oedema pre or post-mating, an oedema pattern that does not extend throughout the uterine wall (Samper, 2009) or the presence of short, thick, hyperechoic lines within the uterine wall signifying either air or exudate. Uterine culture and cytology are common techniques for diagnosis of endometritis, through their respective detection of uterine pathogens and inflammatory cells (neutrophils). If a uterine pathogen is isolated and the mare has more than two neutrophils per 400x field (a positive uterine cytology) she can reliably be diagnosed as having endometritis (Riddle et al., 2007). However, mares may also yield positive uterine cytologies with negative uterine cultures, and vice versa.

Recent work indicates that both of the latter scenarios are associated with endometritis and decreased pregnancy rates (Nielsen et al., 2008). Mares positive for *E. coli*, ≥2 organisms, *S. aureus* and *Pseudomonas spp*. had fewer cytology specimens with >2 neutrophils per 400x field (range 19–33%) than mares positive for *Streptococcus b-haemolytic* or *Klebsiella* (range 50–71.4%). and excessive production of endometrial mucus (Burleson et al., 2010).

To determine the relative importance of culture and cytology, it is helpful to have a 'gold standard' for the presence or absence of disease against which the results can be compared, and thereby generate estimates of sensitivity (per cent of disease-positive which test positive) and specificity (per cent of disease-negative which test negative). With this approach, Nielsen et al., (2008) used the presence of neutrophil infiltration of the luminal epithelium and stratum compactum as a gold standard to indicate the presence of endometritis in 212 uterine biopsies. Against neutrophil infiltration, he compared culture of the endometrial biopsy tissue specimen, swabbing of the endometrium using a guarded culture swab and uterine cytology by smearing the biopsy on a slide. Of the three techniques (biopsy culture, swab culture and cytology), sensitivities were calculated to be 0.82, 0.34 and 0.77, and specificities 0.92, 1.0 and 1.0, respectively (LeBlanc, 2010).

Endometritis can also be influenced by the offending pathogen and the mare's subsequent immunological response to it. Different bacteria express different virulent factors and have different modes of evading the immune response. This can result in an array of clinical signs, ultrasonographic and laboratory findings. Some bacteria such as *Escherichia coli* tenaciously adhere to epithelial surfaces, preventing their physical removal. Others such as streptococci stimulate production of an inflammatory exudate, interfering with neutrophil phagocytosis. *Pseudomonas aeruginosa* and some yeast and fungi secrete a biofilm, an adhesive matrix that supports growth and maintenance of bacterial micro-colonies. Biofilms provide inherent resistance to antibiotics and both celular and humeral immune defences resulting in persistent, chronic infections even after prolonged antibiotic treatment. Some bacteria or fungi form focal plaques that are not identified by routine swab culture techniques, while others do not produce intra-uterine fluid, the 'hallmark' of endometritis. The uterine response to a pathogen also contributes to the establishment and chronicity of infection. During acute and subacute endometritis, mucus production by epitelial cells lining the endometrium, (LeBlanc et al., 2007), is increased; while in chronically inflamed endometria, there is loss of the epithelium and mucus blanket and increased opportunities for bacterial adhesion. Changes in the production, elasticity or viscosity of endometrial mucus can interfere with the ability of the mucociliary apparatus to remove particulate matter, with sperm migrating to the oviduct or with antibiotic penetration by the endometrium. Because of the many factors affecting fertility, clinicians need to tailor their diagnostics specifically for each individual. Recent data indicate that ultrasonographic and cytological findings from mares with endometritis differ between uterine pathogens and that uterine swabs have lower sensitivity in identifying gram-negative organisms than culture of small volume uterine flushings or endometrial biopsy (Causey et al., 2008).

6. High-Risk Pregnant Mare

6.1. Mare Reproductive Loss Syndrome

The maintenance of pregnancy involves a complex interchange of hormonal, biochemical and immunological signals between the mare and the foal (Allen et al., 1987). Embryonic and fetal death in mares is associated with genetic and environmental factors as vaginal infections and uterine abnormalities. This has an impact on premature pregnancy loss by failing to meet the metabolic needs of pregnancy. Irregular and unbalanced nutrition and stress can also cause embryonic end fetal death (Yang and Cho, 2007).

Previous studies have identified differing prevalence and conflicting risk factors for pregnancy losses in Thoroughbred mares. Brück et al., (1993) reported a pregnancy rate of 83.9%, with a pregnancy test done between day 12 and 100 after the date of last service. The foaling rate was 69.3%. The pregnancy rate for mares 3 to 10 years old was significantly higher than for older mares.

No significant difference was found between the pregnancy rates of maiden mares, barren mares or foaling mares. Also the foaling rates were significantly higher for mares 3 to 10 years old than for older mares. Maiden mares had a significantly higher foaling rate than barren or foaling mars. Of all diagnosed pregnancies 19.5 % were lost. In mares aged 3 to 5 years pregnancy loss occurred significantly less than in older mares.

Morris et al., (2007) found a pregnancy rate of 94.8% at day 15 after ovulation, which fell to 89.7% at day 35 after ovulation. Only 5.2% had never been diagnosed pregnant and 17.3 % of the pregnancies diagnosed at around day 15 were subsequently lost. Of those pregnancy losses 59.7% occurred before day 35; 82.7% of the mares gave birth to a life foal at term. The lowest pregnancy rates occurred in mares aged >14 and in mares that were not served the season before. Age had a significant effect on the proportions pregnancies that were lost. Young mares (3 to 8 years old) lost fewer pregnancies before day 35, but they lost more pregnancies after day 35 than older mares (9 to 13). Maiden mares lost fewer pregnancies before day 35. Overall pregnancy lost was highest in mares that aborted the year before.

In Sweden, a small research project by Hemberg et al., (2004) reported a pregnancy rate of 90.9% and a foaling rate of 79.8%. The age of the mare had a significant effect on the foaling rate, but not on the pregnancy rate. Associated with this, the pregnancy loss rate from the first pregnancy diagnosis was the highest in mares older than 13 years. Barren mares and aborted mares showed a significantly higher pregnancy loss rate than maiden and foaling mares.

Yang and Cho (2007) reported a pregnancy rate of 97.9% when pregnancy was confirmed 15 days post ovulation; 12.2% of the mares lost their embryos within 45 days post ovulation. The prevalence of early embryonic death was higher in barren mares (17.2%), mares older than 15 years (15.4%) and mares with a parity higher than 10 (18.2%). The lowest embryonic death rate of 9.8% occurred in mares that experienced abortion or stillbirth during the previous breeding season. Three-quarters of the number of embryonic deaths were detected within 25 days after ovulation, so between day 15 and 26.

More recently, Nath et al., (2010) reported a pregnancy rate of 68.8%, when pregnancy was diagnosed at day 13 and 21 using ultrasound. The highest pregnancy rates were found in maiden mares. Mares 2 to 13 years old had a significantly higher pregnancy rate than mares >13 years old. 7.1% of the mares lost their pregnancy between day 13 and day 45 after ovulation, with the lowest incidence in mares 2 to 8 years old.

Improved diagnostic techniques and advances in the understanding of equine reproductive physiology and pathology have resulted in increased pregnancy rates in mares. In contrast, the incidence of pregnancy loss has remained fairly constant at a rate of 10–15% (Roberts, 1986). Pregnancy losses during late gestation (>5 months) represent an even greater problem for the equine breeding industry. Affected mares will not only fail to produce a foal, but will often have a lower conception rate during the next breeding season. Pregnancy losses during late gestation could be the result of fetal illness, placental dysfunction, or maternal illness. Pre-partum disorders of the mare are easy to diagnose, but identifying conditions that affects the fetus and the placenta may be more difficult. Monitoring of the fetus and the placenta during late gestation is routinely performed in human pregnancies, but has only recently gained recognition in equine veterinary medicine. High risk pregnant mares should be monitored for fetal and placental well-being (Troedsson, 2007).

6.2. Identification of the Compromised Fetus: A Clinical Perspective

Antepartum evaluation of the fetus to assess wellbeing is performed routinely in human obstetric practice. Human infants may be delivered at any stage of the third trimester with a high chance of a successful outcome given good neonatal care facilities. Maturation is stimulated in these infants before induction of parturition by giving the mother betamethasone. At present, this type of treatment protocol does not work in the premature equine fetus. Unlike human infants, viability in the foal is very dependent upon adrenocortical maturation which occurs only near full term, during the last 5 to 7 days of in utero development (gestation length varies from 320 to 360 days in the mare). Viable foals may be born as early as day 290 of gestation if the dam experiences a slowly spreading placental insult such as ascending placentitis. However, some of these foals will have defects in skeletal and other systems serious enough to necessitate euthanasia. Experimental induction of precocious maturation has been investigated but has largely been unsuccessful. Injections of betamethasone or CRF to fetuses between 250 and 310 days of gestation are associated with a rise in maternal progestin concentrations but not the delivery of a precociously mature foal (Rossdale et al., 1992). Repeated injection of adrenocorticotrophic hormone (ACTH) into the fetus at 300 days gestation results in the birth of precociously mature foals but the technique is associated with a high abortion rate. Parturition can be induced successfully by administration of extremely high doses of dexamethasone but such doses have severe deleterious consequences for the mare (Eyre et al., 1979).

Most clinicians feel that the high-risk equine fetus has a better chance of survival if it remains in the uterus, no matter how severely compromised, because early intervention results in the birth of a dysmature foal that will probably die. In the majority of cases this is the correct decision but there are circumstances where it may be better to remove the fetus. Identifying which cases should be induced, and when to intervene, is at best a guess since clinical perinatal medicine is a relatively new discipline in the horse. In the last 5 years, methodologies have been developed to identify the compromised equine fetus. There are few studies, though, on the development of appropriate treatment regimes for the compromised fetus. This paper will discuss clinical assessment of fetal wellbeing and preferred treatment for pregnant mares that are at high risk of fetal loss. It is possible to identify the compromised equine fetus; however, options for treatment and management are severely limited.

Because of these problems some veterinary clincians view antepartum assessment as an exercise in futility. It is unlikely that there will be major advances in clinical perinatal medicine until the endocrine mechanisms that are involved in the control of fetal maturation are identified (Le Blanc, 1997).

References

Ababneh, M., Ababneh, H., Shidaifat, F. (2011). Expression of cytosolic phospholipase A2 in equine endometrium during the oestrous cycle and early pregnancy. *Reprod. Domest. Anim.* 46(2), 268-274.

Abd-Elnaeim, M.M.M., Leiser, R., Wilsher, S., Allen, W.R. (2006). Structural and haemovascular aspects of placental growth throughout gestation in young and aged mares. *Placenta* 27(11), 1103-113.

Abd-Elnaeim, M.M., Derar, I.R., Wilsher, S., Allen, W.R., Leiser, R., Schuler, G. (2009). Immunohistochemical localization of oestrogen receptors alpha and beta, progesterone receptor and aromatase in the equine placenta. *Reprod. Domest. Anim.* 44(2), 312-319.

Al-Katanani, Y.M., Hansen, P.J. (2002). Induced thermotolerance in bovine two-cell embryos and the role of heat shock protein 70 in embryonic development. *Mol. Reprod. Dev.* 62, 174-180.

Allen, W.R. (1969a). A quantitative immunological assay for pregnant mare serum gonadotrophin. *J. Endocrinol.* 43, 581–591.

Allen, W.R. (1969b). Factors influencing pregnant mare serum gonadotrophin production. *Nature* 223, 64–66.

Allen, W.R. (2000). The physiology of early pregnancy in the mare. In: *Proceeding of the 46th Annual Convention of the American Association of Equine Practitioners*, pp. 338-354.

Allen, W.R. (2001a). Fetomaternal interactions and influences during equine pregnancy. *Reproduction* 121, 513–527.

Allen, W.R. (2001b). Luteal deficiency and embryo mortality in the mare. *Reprod. Dom. Anim.* 36, 121-131.

Allen, W.R., Kydd, J.H., Boyle, M.S., Antzak, D.F. (1987). Extraspecific donkey-in-horse pregnancy as a model of early fetal death. *J. Reprod. Fertil. Suppl.* 35, 197–209.

Allen, W.R., Brown, L., Wright, M., Wilsher, S. (2007). Reproductive efficiency of Thoroughbred Flatrace and National Hunt mares and stallions in England. *Equine Vet. J.* 29, 338-345.

Allen, W.R., Stewart, F. (2001). Equine placentation. *Reprod. Fertil. Dev,* 13, 623-634.

Allen, W.R., Wilsher, S., Turnbull, C., Stewart, F., Ousey, J., Rossdale, P.D., Fowden, A.L. (2002). Influence of maternal size on placental, fetal and postnatal growth in the horse. I. Development in utero. *Reproduction* 123, 445-453.

Allen, W.R., Wilsher, S. (2009). A review of implantation and early placentation in the mare. *Placenta* 30, 1005-1015.

Arar, S., Chan, K.H., Quinn, B.A., Waelchli, R.O., Hayes, M.A., Betteridge, K.J. (2007). Desialylation of core type 1 O-glycan in the equine embryonic capsule coincides with immobilization of the conceptus in the uterus. *Carb. Res.* 342, 1110-1115.

Asa, C.S., Ginther, O.J. (1982). Glucocorticoid suppression of estrous, follicles, LH, and ovulation in the mare. *J. Reprod. Fertil. Suppl.* 32, 247-251.

Bae, S. E., and Watson, E. D. (2003). A light microscopic and ultrastructural study on the presence and location of oxytocin in the equine endometrium. *Theriogenology* 60, 909–921.

Baker, C., Adams, M.H., McDowell, K.J. (1991). Lack of expression of alpha or omega interferons by the horse conceptus. *J. Reprod. Fertil. Suppl.* 44, 439-443.

Ball, B.A. (1988). Embryonic loss in mares. Incidence, possible causes, and diagnostic considerations. *Vet. Clin. North Am. Equine Pract.* 4, 263–290.

Ball, B. A. (1993). Embryonic death in mares. *In: Equine Reproduction,* (McKinnon, A.O., Voss, J.L., Eds.). Lea & Febiger, Philadelphia, pp. 517–531.

Ball, B.A., Miller, P.G. (1992). Survival of equine embryos co-cultured with equine oviductal epithelium from the four- to eight-cell to the blastocyst stage after transfer to synchronous recipient mares. *Theriogenology* 37, 979–991.

Battut, I., Grandchamp, A., Nicaise, J.L., Fieni, F., Tanturier, D., Bruyas, J.F. (2001). When do equine embryos enter the uterine cavity? An attempt to answer. *In: Proceedings of the 5th Internacional Symposium on Equine Embryo Transfer.* Newmarket: R&W Publications, pp. 66-68.

Baucus, K.L., Squires, E.L., Ralston, S.L., McKinnon, A.O., Nett, T.M. (1990). Effect of transportation on the estrous cycle and concentrations of hormones in mare. *J. Anim. Sci,* 68, 419-426.

Bazer, F.W., Ott, T.L., Spencer, T.E. (1998). Endocrinology of the transition from recurring estrous cycles to establishment of pregnancy in sub-primate mammals. *In: The Endocrinology of Pregnancy.* (Bazer, F.W. Ed.). Humana Press Inc., Totowa, NJ.

Beckelmann, J., Budik, S., Helmreich, M., Palm, F., Walter, I., Aurich, C. (2013). Sex-dependent insulin like growth factor-1 expression in preattachment equine embryos. *Theriogenology* 79(1), 193-199.

Bergfelt, D.R., Pierson, R.A., Ginther, O.J. (1989). Resurgence of the primary corpus luteum during pregnancy in the mare. *Anim. Reprod. Sci.* 21, 261–270.

Bergfelt, D.R., Woods, J.A., Ginther, O.J. (1992). Role of the embryonic vesicle and progesterone in embryonic loss in mares. *J. Reprod. Fertil.* 1(95), 339–347.

Bergfelt, D.R., Ginther, O.J. (1996). Ovarian, uterine and embryodynamics in horses versus ponies. *J. Equine Vet. Sci.* 16, 66–72.

Berglund, L.A., Sharp, D.C., Vernon, M.W., Thatcher, W.W. (1982). Effect of pregnancy and collection technique on prostaglandin F in the uterine lumen of Pony mares. *J. Reprod. Fertil. Suppl.* 32, 335-341.

Betancourt-Alonso, M.A., Flores-Perez, F.I., Rosas-Velasco, C., Perez-Martinez, C. (2006). Role of cytokines in embryo implantation in domestic mammals. *Vet. Mex.* 37, 335–350.

Betteridge, K.J., Eaglesome, M.D., Mitchell, D., Flood, P.F., Beriault, R. (1982). Development of horse embryos up to twenty two days after ovulation: observation of fresh specimens. *J. Anat.* 135(1), 191-209.

Betteridge, K.J. (1989). Structure and function of the equine capsule in relation to embryo manipulation and transfer. *Equine Vet. J. Suppl.* 8, 92–100.

Betteridge, K,J. (2000). Comparative aspects of equine embryonic development. *Anim. Reprod. Sci.* 60, 691-702.

Betteridge, K.J. (2007). Equine embryology: an inventory of unanswered questions. *Theriogenology* 1(68), 9-21.

Betteridge, K.J. (2011). Embryo morphology, growth and development. *In: Equine Reproduction.* (Mckinnon, A.O., Squires, E.L., Vaala, W.E., Varner, D.D. Eds.). Willey-Blackwell, pp. 2167-2186.

Betteridge, K.J., Waelchli, R.O., Christie, H.L., Raeside, J.I., Quinn, B.A., Hayes, M.A. (2012). Relationship between the timing of prostaglandin-induced luteolysis and effects on the conceptus during early pregnancy in mares. *Reprod Fertil Dev.* 24(3), 411-424.

Biggers, B.G., Geisert, R.D., Wetteman, R.P., Buchanan, D.S. (1987). Effect of heat stress on early embryonic development in the beef cow. *J. Anim. Sci.* 64, 1512-1518.

Blanchard, T.L., Thompson, J.A., Brinsko, S.P., Stick, K.L., Wendt, K.M., Varner, D.D., Rigby, S.L. (2004). Mating mares on foal heat: a five year retrospective study. In: *Proceedings of the 50th Annual Convention of the American Association of Equine Practitioners*, pp. 525–530.

Boerboom, D., Brown, K.A., Vaillancourt, D., Poitras, P., Goff, A.K., Watanabe, K., Dore, M., Sirois, J. (2004). Expression of key prostaglandin synthases in equine endometrium during late diestrus and early pregnancy. *Biol. Reprod.* 70, 391-399.

Bollwein, H., Woschee, I., Stolla, R. (1999). Uterine durchblutung wahrend der graviditat der stute. *Pferdeheilkunde* 15, 595-598.

Bonafos, L.D., Carnevale, E.M., Smith, C.A., Ginther, O.J. (1994). Development of uterine tone in nonbred and pregnant mares. *Theriogenology* 42, 1247–1255.

Bracher, V., Mathias, S., Allen, W.R. (1996). Influence of chronic degenerative endometritis (endometrosis) on placental development in the mare. *Equine Vet. J.* 28, 180-188.

Brandt, Y., Einarsson, S., Ljung, A., Lundeheim, N., Rodríguez-Martínez, H., Madej, A. (2009). Effects of continuous elevated cortisol concentrations during estrus on concentrations and patterns of progesterone, oestradiol and LH in the sow. *Anim. Reprod. Sci.* 110, 172-185.

Brinsko, S.P., Ball, B.A., Ignotz, G.G., Thomas, P.G.A., Currie, W, B., Ellington, J.E. (1995). Initiation of transcription and nucleogenesis in equine embryos. *Mol. Reprod. Dev.* 42, 298-302.

Brinsko, S.P., Rigby, S.L., Varner, D.D., Blanchard, J.L. (2003). A practical method for recognizing mares susceptible to post-breeding endometritis. In: *Proceeding of American Association of Equine Practitioners,* 49, 363–365.

Brück, I., Anderson, G.A., Hyland, J. H. (1993). Reproductive performance of Thoroughbred mares on six commercial stud farms. *Aust. Vet. J.* 70, 299-303.

Bucca, S., Carli, A., Buckley, T., Dolci, G., Fogarty, U. (2008). The use of dexamethasone administered to mares at breeding time in the modulation of persistent mating induced endometritis. *Theriogenology* 70, 1093–1100.

Budik, S., Lussy, H., Aurich, C. (2010). Quantification of different type I interferons in equine embryos at days 10–16 of gestation. *Anim. Reprod. Sci.* 121, 307–308.

Budik, S., Palm, F., Walter, I., Helmreich, M., Aurich, C. (2012). Increasing expression of oxytocin and vasopressin receptors in the equine conceptus between Days 10 and 16 of pregnancy. *Reprod. Fertil. Dev.* 24(5), 641-648.

Burleson, M.D., LeBlanc, M.M., Riddle, W.T., Hendricks, K.E.M. (2010). Endometrial microbial isolates are associated with different ultrasonographic and endometrial cytology findings in Thoroughbred mares. In: *Proceedings International Symposium on Equine Reproduction*. Wiley-Blackwell, Lexington, KY.

Burns, P. D., Graf, G. A., Hayes, S. H., and Silvia, W. J. (1997). Cellular mechanisms by which oxytocin stimulates uterine PGF2 alpha synthesis in bovine endometrium: roles of phospholipases C and A2. *Domest. Anim. Endocrinol.* 14, 181–191.

Carnevale, E.M., Ginther, O.J. (1992). Relationships of age to reproductive function and uterine efficiency in mares. *Theriogenology* 237, 1101-1115.

Carnevale, E.M., Griffin, P.G., Ginther, O.J. (1993). Age-associated subfertility before entry of embryos into the uterus of the mare. *Equine Vet. J. Suppl.* 15, 31–35.

Carnevale, E.M., Ramirez, R.J., Squires, E.L., Alvarenga, M.A., Vanderwall, D.K., McCue, P.M. (2000). Factors affecting pregnancy rates and early embrionic death after equine embryo transfer. *Theriogenology* 54(6), 965-979.

Causey, R.C., Miletello, T., O'Donnell, L., Lyle, S.K., Paccamonti, D.L., Anderson, K.J., Eilts, B.E., Morse, S., LeBlanc, M.M. (2008). Pathologic effects of clinical uterine inflammation on the equine endometrial mucosa. In: *Proceeding of American Association of Equine Practitioners*, 54, 276–277.

Chaney, K.P., Holcombe, S.J., LeBlanc, M.M., Hauptman, J.G., Embertson, R.M.,Mueller, P.O.E., Beard, W.L. (2006). Effect of uterine torsion on mare and foal survival: a retrospective study 1985–2005. In: *Proceeding of American Association of Equine Practitioner,* 52, 402-403.

Chavatte, P., Holtan, D.W., Ousey, J.C. and Rossdale, P.D. (1997). Biosynthesis and possible biological role of progestagens during equine pregnancy and in the newborn foal. *Equine Vet. J. Suppl.* 24, 89–95.

Christiansen, D., Crouch, J., Hopper, R., Moulton, K., LeBlanc, M.M., Ryan, P.L. (2009). Experimentally induced placentitis in late gestation mares with *Streptococcus equi zooepidemicus*: therapeutic prevention of preterm birth. *Clin. Theriogenol.* 1, 239.

Chu, J.W., Sharon, F.J., Oriol, J.G., Betteridge, K.J., Cleaver, B.D., Sharp, D.C. (1997). Biochemical changes in the equine capsule following prostaglandin-induced pregnancy failure. *Mol. Reprod. Dev.* 46(3), 286-295.

Cochet, M., Vaiman, D., Lefevre, F. (2009). Novel interferon delta genes in mammals: cloning of one gene from the sheep, two genes expressed by the horse conceptus and discovery of related sequences in several taxa by genomic database screening. *Gene* 433, 88-99.

Coignoul, F.L., Cheville, N.F. (1984). Pathology of maternal genital tract, placenta, and fetus in equine viral arteritis. *Vet. Pathol.* 21, 333-340.

Cooke, R. G., and Ahmad, N. (1994). Prostaglandin E2 alpha-induced release of oxytocin from ovine corpora lutea in vitro. *Prostaglandins* 48, 257–261.

Coss, R.A., Linnemans, W.A.M. (1996). The effects of hyperthermia on the cytoskeleton: a review. *Int. J. Hyperthermia.* 12, 173-196.

Crossett, B., Suire, S., Herrler, A., Allen, W.R., Stewart, F. (1998). Transfer of a uterine lipocalin from the endometrium of the mare to the developing equine conceptus. *Biol. Reprod.* 59, 483-490.

Daher, S., Denardi, K.A.G., Blotta, M.H.S., Mamoni, R.L., Monterio Leck, A.P., Camano, L., Mattar, R. (2004). Cytokines in recurrent pregnancy loss. *J. Reprod. Immunol.* 62, 151–157.

Daley, C.A., Sakurai, H., Adams, B.M., Adams, T.E. (2000). Effect of stress-like concentrations of cortisol on the feedback potency of oestradiol in orchidectomized sheep. *Anim. Reprod. Sci.* 59, 167-178.

Davies Morel, M.C.G., O'Sullivan, J.A.M. (2001). Ovulation rate and distribution in the Thoroughbred mare, as determined by ultrasonic scanning: the effect of age. *Anim. Reprod. Sci.* 66, 59–70.

Davies Morel, M.C.G., Newcombe, J., Swindlehurst, J. (2005). The effect of age on multiple ovulation rates, multiple pregnancy rates and embryonic vesicle diameter in the mare. *Theriogenology* 63(9), 2482-2493.

Davies Morel, M.C.G., Newcombe, J.R., Hinchliffe, J. (2009). The relationship between consecutive pregnancies in Thoroughbred mares. Does the location of one pregnancy affect the location of the next, is this affected by mare age and foal heat to conception interval or related to pregnancy success. *Theriogenology* 71, 1072–1078.

Denker, H.W. (2000). Structural dynamics and function of early embryonic coats. *Cell Tiss. Org.* 166(2), 180-207.

Dziuk, P. (1985). Effect of migration, distribution and spacing of pig embryos on pregnancy and fetal survival. *J. Reprod. Fertil. Suppl.* 33, 57-63.

Ealy, A.D., Arechiga, C.F., Bray, D.R., Risco, C.A., Hansen, P.J. (1994). Effectiveness of short-term cooling and vitamin E for alleviation of infertility induced by heat stress in dairy cows. *J. Dairy Sci.* 77, 3601-3607.

Ealy, A.D., Eroh, M.L., Sharp, D.C. III. (2010). Prostaglandin H synthase Type 2 is differentially expressed in endometrium based on pregnancy status in pony mares and responds to oxytocin and conceptus secretions in explant culture. *Anim. Reprod. Sci. 117,* 99-105.

Ellenberger, C., Wilsher, S., Allen, W.R., Hoffmann, C., Kolling, M., Bazer, F.W., Klug, J., Schoon, D., Schoon, H.A. (2008). Immunolocalisation of the uterine secretory proteins uterocalin, uteroferrin and uteroglobin in the mare's uterus and placenta throughout pregnancy. *Theriogenology* 70, 746-757.

Enders, A.C., Lantz, K.C., Liu, I.K.M., Schlafke, S. (1988). Loss of polar trophoblast during differentiation of the blastocyst of the horse. *J. Reprod. Fertil.* 83(1), 447-460.

Enders, A.C., Liu, I.K. (1991). Lodgement of the equine blastocyst in the uterus from fixation through endometrial cup formation. *J. Reprod. Fertil. Suppl.* 44, 427-438.

Enders, A.C., Schlafke, S., Lantz, K.C. & Liu, I.K. (1993). Endoderm cells of the equine yolk sac from day 7 until formation of the definitive yolk sac placenta. *Equine Vet. J.* 25(15), 3-9.

Eyre, P., Elmes, P.J., Strickland, S. (1979). Corticosteroid-potentiated vascular responses of the equine digit: a possible pharmacologic basis for laminitis. *Am. J. Vet. Res.* 40, 135-138.

Ezzo, O.H., Amal, A.A., Abo El-Maaty, A.M., Mahmoud, K.G.M. (2011). Hormonal and Cytogenetic Investigations in Mares with Early Embryonic Death. *Global Vet.* 7(3), 211-218.

Fairclough, R. J., Moore, L. G., McGowan, L. T., Peterson, A. J., Smith, J. F., Tervit, H. R., Watkins, W. B. (1980). Temporal relationship between plasma concentrations of 13, 14-dihydro-15-keto-prostaglandin F and neurophysin I/II around luteolysis in sheep. *Prostaglandins* 20, 199–208.

Ferreira, J.C., Gastal, E.L., Ginther, O.J. (2008). Uterine blood flow and perfusion in mares with uterine cysts: effect of size of the cystic area and age. *Reproduction* 135, 541-550.

Forsey, K.E., Ellis, P.J., Sargent, C.A., Sturmey, R.G., Leese, H.J. (2013). Expression and localization of creatine kinase in the preimplantation embryo. *Mol. Reprod. Dev.* 80(3), 185-192.

Franciolli, A.L., Cordeiro, B.M., da Fonseca, E.T., Rodrigues, M.N., Sarmento, C.A., Ambrosio, C.E., de Carvalho, A.F., Miglino, M.A., Silva, L.A. (2011). Characteristics of the equine embryo and fetus from days 15 to 107 of pregnancy. *Theriogenology* 76(5), 819-832.

Frazer, G. (2011). Dystocie management. *In: Equine Reproduction.* (Mckinnon, A.O., Squires, E.L., Vaala, W.E., Varner, D.D., Eds.). Willey-Blackwell, pp. 2479-2498.

Gaivão, M., Stout, T. (2012). Equine conceptus development – A mini review. *Revista Lusófona de Ciência e Medicina Veterinária* 5, 64-72.

Gastal, M.O., Gastal, E.L., Kot, K., Ginther, O.J. (1996). Factors related to the time of fixation of the conceptus in mares. *Theriogenology* 46, 1171–1180.

Gastal, M.O., Gastal, E.L., Torres, C.A.A., Ginther, O.J. (1998). Effect of PGE2 on uterine contractility and tone in mares. *Theriogenology* 50(7), 989-999.

Gilbert, R.O., Marlow, C.H.B. (1992). A field study of patterns of unobserved foetal less as determined by rectal palpation in foaling, barren and maiden Thoroughbred mares. *Equine Vet. J.* 24, 184–186.

Gilbert, S.F. (2000). Early embryonic development. *In*: *Developmental Biology* (Gilbert, F.L. Ed.), Sunderland: Sinauer Associates, pp. 185-373.

Giles, R.C., Donahue, J.M., Hong, C.B., Tuttle, P.A., Petrites-Murphy, M.B., Poonacha, K.B., Roberts, A.W., Tramontin, R.R., Smith, B., Swerczek, T.W. (1993). Causes of abortion, stillbirth, and perinatal death in horses: 3,527 cases (1986-1991). *J. Am. Vet. Med. Assoc.* 203, 1170–1175.

Ginther, O.J. (1981). Local versus systemic uteroovarian relationships in farm animals. *Acta Vet. Scand. Suppl.* 77, 103–115.

Ginther, O.J. (1983,a). Mobility of the early equine conceptus. *Theriogenology*19(4), 603-611.

Ginther, O.J. (1983,b). Fixation and orientation of the early equine conceptus. *Theriogenology* 19(4), 613-623.

Ginther, O.J. (1985). Dynamic physical interactions between equine embryo and uterus. *Equine Vet. J. Suppl.* 3, 41–47.

Ginther, O.J. (1985). Embryonic loss in mares: nature of loss after experimental induction by ovariectomy or prostaglandin F2a. *Theriogenology* 24, 87-98.

Ginther, O.J. (1986). The single embryo. In: *Ultrasonic imaging and reproductive events in the mare*. Cross Plains, Wis: Equiservices, pp. 212–213.

Ginther, O.J. (1989). Twin embryos in mares I: from ovulation to fixation. *Equine Vet. J.* 21, 166–170.

Ginther, O.J. (1992,a). Chapter 9: Embryology and Placentation. *In*: O.J. Ginther (Ed.), *Reproductive biology of the mare* (Gilbert, S.F. Ed.). Cross Plains: Equiservices, pp. 345-418.

Ginther, O.J. (1992,b). Embryology and placentation. In: *Reproductive biology of the mare: basic and applied aspects*. Cross Plains, Wis: Equiservices, pp. 350–351.

Ginther, O.J. (1993). Equine fetal kinetics: Allantoic-fluid shifts and uterine-horn closures. *Theriogenology* 40, 241–256.

Ginther, O.J. (1995). Embryo. *In: Ultrasonic Imaging and Animal Reproduction: Horses*. (Ginther, O.J. Ed.). Cross Plains WI: Equiservices, pp: 123-155.

Ginther, O.J. (1998) Equine Pregnancy: Physical interactions between the uterus and conceptus. *Proceeding of American Association of Equine Practitioners* 44, 73-104.

Ginther, O.J., Williams, D., Curran, S. (1994). Equine fetal kinetics: Entry and retention of fetal hind limbs in a uterine horn. *Theriogenology* 41, 795–807.

Givens, M.D., Marley, M.S. (2008). Infectious causes of embryonic and fetal mortality. *Theriogenology* 70(3), 270-285.

Goff, A.K. (2002). Embryonic signals and survival. *Reprod. Domest. Anim.* 37(1), 133-139.

Goff, A.K., Leduc, S., Poitras, P., Vaillancourt, D. (1993). Steroid synthesis by equine conceptuses between days 7 and 14 and endometrial steroid metabolism. *Domest. Anim. Endocrinol.* 10, 229–236.

Gravett, M.G., Hitti, J., Hess, D.L., Eschenbach, D.A. (2000). Intrauterine infection and preterm delivery: evidence for activation of the fetal hypothalamic-pituitary-adrenal axis. *Am. J. Obstet. Gynecol.* 182, 1404-1410.

Green, J.A., Xie, S., Szafranska, B., Gan, X., Newman, A.G., McDowell, K., Roberts, R.M. (1999). Identification of a new aspartic proteinase expressed by the outer chorionic layer of the equine placenta. *Biol. Reprod.* 60, 1069–1077.

Griffin, P.G., Ginther, O.J. (1990). Uterine contractile activity in mares during the estrous cycle and early pregnancy. *Theriogenology* 34, 47–56.

Griffin, P.G., Ginther, O.J. (1991a). Dynamics of uterine diameter and endometrial morphology during the estrous cycle and early pregnancy in mares. *Anim. Reprod. Sci.* 25, 133–142.

Griffin, P.G., Ginther, O.J. (1991b). Uterine morphology and function in postpartum mares. *J. Equine Vet. Sci.* 11, 330–339.

Griffin, P.G., Ginther, O.J. (1993). Effects of the embryo on uterine morphology and function in mares. *Anim. Reprod. Sci.* 31, 311–329.

Grøndahl, C., Grøndahl Nielsen, C., Eriksen, T., Greve, T., Hyttel, P. (1993). In-vivo fertilisation and initial embryogenesis in the mare. *Equine Vet. J. Suppl.* 15, 79–83.

Hafez, E.S.E., Hafez, B. (2000). Fertilization and Cleavage. *In: Reproduction in Farm Animals* (Hafez, E.S.E., Hafez, B. Ed.). New York: Wiley-Blackwell, pp. 110-125.

Hamon, M., Clarke, S.W., Houghton, E., Fowden, A.L., Silver, M., Rossdale, P.D., Ousey, J.C., Heap, R.B. (1991). Production of 5 –dihydro-progesterone during late pregnancy in the mare. *J. Reprod. Fertil. Suppl.* 44, 529–535.

Hansen, P.J., Drost, M., Rivera, R.M., Paula-Lopes, F.F., Al-Katanani, Y.M., Krininger III, C.E., Chase Jr. C.C. (2001). Adverse impact on heat stress on embryo production: Causes and strategies for mitigation. *Theriogenology* 55, 91-103.

Hayes, M.A., Quinn, B.A., Lillie, B.N., Côté, O., Bienzle, D., Waelchli, R.O., Betteridge, K.J. (2012). Changes in various endometrial proteins during cloprostenol-induced failure of early pregnancy in mares. *Anim. Reprod.* 9(4), 723-741.

Hemberg, E., Lundeheim, N., Einarsson, S. (2004). Reproductive performance of Thoroughbred mares in Sweden. *Reprod. Domest. Anim.* 39(2), 81-85.

Herrler, A., Stewart, F., Allen, W.R., Beier, H.M. (1999). Proteins detectable in the coats of preimplantation rabbit and horse embryos. *J. Reprod. Fertil. Abstr. Ser.* 23, 80.

Herrler, A., Beier, H.M. (2000). Early embryonic coats: morphology, function, practical applications. *Cell Tiss. Org.* 166, 233–246.

Herrler, A., Pell, J.M., Allen, W.R., Beier, H.M., Stewart, F. (2000). Horse conceptuses secrete insulin-like growth factor-binding protein 3. *Biol. Reprod.* 62(6), 1804-1811.

Herrler, A., Stewart, F., Crossett, B., Pell, J.M., Ellis, P.D., Brown, K.D., Beier, H.M., Allen, W.R. (1998). Maternal and embryonic proteins in the equine blastocyst capsule. *In: Proceeding of 7th International Symposium of Equine Reproduction,* Pretoria, pp: 157–158.

Hicks, B.A., Etter, S.J., Carnahan, K.G., Joyce, M.M., Assiri, A.A., Carlin, S.J., Kodali, K., Johnson, G.A., Hansen, T.R., Mirando, M.A., Woods, G.L., Vanderwall, D.K., Ott, T.L. (2003). Expression of the uterine Mx protein in cyclic and pregnant cows, gilts, and mares. *J. Anim. Sci.* 81, 1552-1561.

Holtan, D.W., Nett, T.M., Estergreen, V.L. (1975). Plasma progestagens in pregnant mares. *J. Repod. Fertil. Suppl.* 23, 419-424.

Holtan, D.W., Houghton, E., Silver, M., Fowden, A.L. Ousey, J., Rossdale, P.D. (1991). Plasma progestagens in the mare fetus and newborn foal. *J. Reprod. Fertil. Suppl.* 44, 517–528.

Hong, C.B., Donahue, J.M., Giles, R.C. Petrites-Murphy, M.B., Poonacha, K.B., Roberts, A.W., Smith, B.J., Tramontin, R.R., Tuttle, P.A., Swerczek, T.W. (1993a). Etiology and pathology of equine placentitis. *J. Vet. Diagn. Invest.* 5, 56–63.

Hunter RH, 2012: Components of oviduct physiology in eutherian mammals. *Biol. Rev. Camb. Philos. Soc.* 87, 244–255.

Hwang, D.H., Pool, S.H., Rorie, R.W., Boudreau, M., Godke, R.A. (1988). Transitional changes in arachidonic acid metabolism by bovine embryos at different developmental stages. *Prostaglandins* 35, 387.

Ingraham, R.H., Gillette, D.D., Wagner, W.D. (1974). Relationship of temperature and humidity to conception rate of Holstein cows in subtropical climate. *J. Dairy Sci.* 57, 476-481.

Irvine, C.H.G., Sutton, P., Turner, J.E., Mennick, P.E. (1990). Changes in plasma progesterone concentrations from days 17 to 42 of gestation in mares maintaining or losing pregnancy. *Equine Vet. J.* 11, 104-106.

Jonker, F.H. (2004). Fetal death: comparative aspects in large domestic animals. *Anim. Reprod. Sci.* 82–83, 415–430.

Kalantaridou, S.N., Makrigiannakis, A., Zoumakis, E., Chrousos, G.P. (2004). Stress and the female reproductive system. *J. Reprod. Immunol.* 62, 61-68.

Katila, T. (2011). Maternal recognition of pregnancy in the horse. *Pferdeheilkunde* 27(3), 261-264.

Kennedy, M.W. (2004) Uterocalin – provider of essential lipids and amino acids to the preplacentation equine conceptus. *In: Havemeyer Foundation Monograph* series 16, pp: 53-56.

Kerbler, T.L., Buhr, M.M., Jordan, L.T., Leslie, K.E., Walton, J.S. (1997). Relationship between maternal plasma progesterone concentration and interferon-tau synthesis by the conceptus in cattle. *Theriogeneology* 47, 703-714.

Klein, C., Troedsson, M.H. (2011). Transcriptional profiling of equine conceptuses reveals new aspects of embryo-maternal communication in the horse. *Biol. Reprod.* 84, 872–885.

Klonisch, T., Mathias, S., Cambridge, G., Hombach-Klonisch, S., Ryan, P.L., Allen, W.R. (1997). Placental localization of relaxin in the pregnant mare. *Placenta* 18, 121–128.

Kölle, S., Dubois, C.S., Caillaud, M., Lahuec, C., Sinowatz, F., Goudet, G. (2007). Equine zona protein synthesis and ZP structure during folliculogenesis, oocyte maturation, and embryogenesis. *Mol. Reprod. Dev.* 74(7), 851-859.

Krakowski, L., Krawczyk, C.H., Wrona, Z., Dabrowski, R., Jarosz, Ł. (2010). Levels of selected T lymphocyte subpopulations in peripheral blood of mares which experienced early embryonic death. *Anim. Reprod. Sci.* 120(1-4), 71-77.

LeBlanc, M.M. (1997). Identification and treatment of the compromised equine fetus: a clinical perspective. *Equine Vet. J., Suppl.* 24, 100-103.

LeBlanc, M.M., Causey, R.C. (2009) Clinical and subclinical endometritis in the mare: both threats to fertility. *Reprod. Domest. Anim.* 44(3), 10–22.

LeBlanc, M.M. (2010). Ascending placentitis in the mare: en update. *Reprod. Dom. Anim.* 45(2), 28–34.

LeBlanc, M.M., Macpherson, M.L., Sheerin, P.C. (2004). Ascending placentitis: what we know about pathophysiology, diagnosis, and treatment. In: *Proceedings of the American Association of Equine Practitioners,* pp. 127–143.

LeBlanc, M.M., Magsig, J., Stromberg, A.J. (2007). Use of a low volume uterine flush for diagnosing endometritis in chronically infertile mares. *Theriogenology* 68, 403–412.

Lechniak, D., Pers-Kamczyc, E., Pawlak, P. (2008). Timing of the first zygotic cleavage as a marker of developmental potential of mammalian embryos. *Reprod. Biol.* 8, 23-42.

Legrand, E., J. M. Krawiecki, D. Tainturier, and J. F. Bruyas. (2001). Does the embryonic capsule impede freezing of equine embryos?. *In: Proceedings of the 5th Internation Symposium on Equine Embryo Transfer*, pp. 62-65.

Legrand, E., Bencharif, D., Barrier-Battut, I., Delajarraud, H., Cornière, P., Fiéni, F., Tainturier, D., Bruyas, J.F. (2002). Comparision of pregnancy rates for days 7-8 equine embryos frozen in glycerol with or without previous enzymatic treatment of their capsule. *Theriogenology* 58, 721-723.

Leiser, R., Pfarrer, C., Adb-Elnaeim, M., Dantzer, V. (1998). Feto-maternal exchange in epitheliochorial placental types studied by histology and microvascular corrosion casts. *Troph. Res.* 12, 21-39.

Leith, G.S., Ginther, O.J. (1984). Characterization of intrauterine mobility of the early conceptus. *Theriogenology* 22(4), 401-408.

Lenz, R.W., Ball, G.D., Leibfried, M.L., Ax, R.L., First, N.L. (1983). In vitro maturation and fertilization of bovine oocytes are temperature-dependent processes. *Biol. Reprod.* 29, 173-179.

Macpherson, M.L. (2006). Diagnosis and treatment of equine placentitis. *Vet. Clin. Equine* 22, 763-776.

Macpherson, C.S., Bailey, C.S. (2008). A clinical approach to managing the mare with placentitis. *Theriogenology* 70, 435–440.

Madic, J., Hajsig, D., Sostaric, B., Curic, S., Seol, B., Naglic, T. (1997). An outbreak of abortion in mares associated with *Salmonella abortus equi* infection. *Equine Vet. J.* 29, 230–233.

Marenzoni, M.L., Lepri, E., Casagrande, P., Bietta, A., Coletti, M., Timoney, P.J., Passamonti, F. (2012). Causes of equine abortion, stillbirth and neonatal death in central Italy. *Vet Rec.* 170(10), 262.

Mastorakos, G., Pavlatou, M., Diamanti-Kandarakis, E., Chrousos, G.P. (2005). Exercise and the stress system. *Hormones* 4(2), 73-89.

Mays, M.B.C., LeBlanc, M.M., Paccamonti, D. (2002). Route of fetal infection in a model of ascending placentitis. *Theriogenology* 58, 791-792.

McCutcheon, L.J., Geor, R.J. (2000). Influence of training on sweating responses during submaximal exercise in horses. *J. Appl. Physiol.* 89, 2463-2471.

McDowell, K.J., Sharp, D.C. (2011). Maternal recognition of pregnancy. In: *Equine Reproduction*. (McKinnon A. O., Squires E. L., Vaala W. E., Varner D. D. Eds). Wiley-Blackwell, U.K., pp. 2200-2210.

McDowell, K.J., Sharp, D.C., Fazleabas, A.T., Roberts, R.M. (1990). Two-dimensional polyacrylamide gel electrophoresis of proteins synthesized and released by conceptuses and endometria from pony mares. *J. Reprod. Fertil.* 89, 107–115.

McDowell, K.J., Sharp, D.C., Grubaugh, W., Thatcher, W.W., Wilcox, C.J. (1988). Restricted conceptus mobility results in failure of pregnancy maintenance in mares. *Biol. Reprod.* 39(2), 340-348.

McKeever, K.H. (2002). The endocrine system and challenge of exercise. *Vet. Clin. Equine* 18, 321-353.

McKinnon, A.O., Lescun, T.B., Walker, J.H., Vasey, J.R., Allen, W.R. (2000). The inability of some synthetic progestagens to maintain pregnancy in the mare. *Equine Vet. J.* 32, 83-85.

McMullen, S., Osgerby, J.C., Milne, J.S., Wallace, J.M., Wathes, D.C. (2005). The effects of acute nutrient restriction in the mid-gestational ewe on maternal and fetal nutrient status, expression of placental growth factors and fetal growth. *Placenta* 26, 25-33.

Merkl, M., Ulbrich, S.E., Otzdorff, C., Herbach, N., Wanke, R., Wolf, E., Handler, J., Bauersachs, S. (2010). Microarray analysis of equine endometrium at days 8 and 12 of pregnancy. *Biol. Reprod.* 83(5), 874-886.

Mihm, M.N., Curran, P., Hyttel, P.G., Knight, M.P., Boland, M., Roche, J.F. (1999). Effects of dominant follicle persistence on follicular fluid oestradiol and inhibin and on oocyte maturation in heifers. *J. Reprod. Fertil. Suppl.* 116, 293-304.

Morley, P.S., Townsend, H.H.G. (1997). A survey of reproductive performance in Thoroughbred mares and morbidity, mortality and athletic potential of their foals. *Equine Vet. J.* 29, 290-297.

Morris, L.H., Allen, W.R. (2002). Reproductive efficiency of intensively managed Thoroughbred mares in Newmarket. *Equine Vet. J.* 34, 51–60.

Morris, S., Kelleman, A.A., Stawicki, R.J., Hansen, P.J., Sheerin, P.C., Sheerin, B.R., Paccamenonti, D.L., LeBlanc, M.M. (2007). Transrectal ultrasonography and plasmaprogestin profiles identifies feto-placental compromise in mares with experimentally induced placentitis. *Theriogenology* 67, 681–691.

Mortensen, C.J. (2007). Effects of exercise or oocyte heat shock on embryo development and gene expression in the horse. PhD Thesis Texas A&M University.

Mortensen, C., Choi, Y., Hinrichs, K., Ing, N., Kraemer, D., Vogelsang, S., Vogelsang, M. (2009). Embryo recovery from exercised mares. *Anim. Reprod. Sci.* 110, 237-244.

Nath, L.C., Anderson, G.A., McKinnon, A.O. (2010). Reproductive efficiency of Thoroughbred and Standardbred horses in north-east Victoria. *Aust. Vet. J.* 88, 169-175.

Needleman, P., Turk, J., Jakschik, B.A., Morrison, A.R., Lefkowith, J.B. (1986). Arachidonic acid metabolism. *Annu. Rev. Biochem.* 55, 69-102.

Newcombe, J.R. (2000). Embryonic loss and abnormalities of early pregnancy. *Equine Vet. Educ.* 2, 115–130.

Nielsen, J.M. (2008). Endometritis in the mare: a diagnostic study comparing cultures from swab and biopsy. *Theriogenology* 64, 510–518.

Oriol, J.G., Sharom, F.J. & Betteridge, K.J. (1993,a). Developmentally regulated changes in the glycoproteins of the equine embryonic capsule. *J. Reprod. Fertil.* 99(2), 653-664.

Oriol, J.G., Betteridge, K.J., Clarke, A.J., Sharom, F.J. (1993,b). Mucin-like glycoproteins in the equine embryonic capsule. *Mol. Reprod. Dev.* 34(3), 255-265.

Ousey, J.C. (2004). Peripartal endocrinology in the mare and foetus. *Reprod. Domest. Anim.* 39, 222–231.

Ousey, J.C., Houghton, E., Grainger, L., Rossdale, P.D., Fowden, A.L. (2005). Progestagen profiles during the last trimester of gestation in Thoroughbred mares with normal or compromised pregnancies. *Theriogenology* 63, 1844–1856.

Ousey, J.C., Kolling, M., Allen, W.R. (2006). The effecs of maternal dexamethasone treatment on gestation length and foal maturation in Thoroughbred mares. *Anim. Reprod. Sci.* 94, 436–438.

Ousey, J.C., Fowden, A.L., Wilsher, S., Allen, W.R. (2008). The effects of maternal health and body condition on the endocrine responses of neonatal foals. *Equine Vet. J.* 40(7), 673-679.

Panzani, S., Castagnetti, C., Prandi, A., Faustini, M., Zamboni, A., Veronesi, M.C. (2013). Insulin-like growth factor I: could it be a marker of prematurity in the foal?. *Theriogenology* 79(3), 495-501.

Papa, F.O., Lopes, M.D., Alvarenga, M.A., Meira, C., Luvizotto, M.C., Ribeiro, E.F., Azedo, A.E., Bomfim, A.C. (1998). Early embryonic death in mares: clinical and hormonal aspects. *Brazilian J. Vet. Res. Anim. Sci.* 35, 170-173.

Pereira, G.R., Lorenzo, P.L., Carneiro, G.F., Ball, B.A., Pegoraro, L.M., Pimentel, C.A., Liu, I.K. (2013). Influence of equine growth hormone, insulin-like growth factor-I and its interaction with gonadotropins on in vitro maturation and cytoskeleton morphology in equine oocytes. *Animal* 7(9), 1493-1499.

Piccinni, M., Scaletti, C., Maggi, E., Romagnani, S. (2000). Role of hormonecontrolled Th1 and Th2 type cytokines in successful pregnancy. *J. Neuroimmunol.* 109, 30–33.

Pontzer, C.H., Bazer, F.W., Johnson, H.M. (1991). Antiproliferative activity of a pregnancy recognition hormone, ovine trophoblast protein-1. *Cancer Res.* 51, 5304-5307.

Pontzer, C.H., Torres, B.A., Vallet, J.L., Bazer, F.W., Johnson, H.M. (1988). Antiviral activity of the pregnancy recognition hormone ovine trophoblast protein-1. *Biochem. Biophys. Res. Commun.* 152, 801-807.

Pool-Anderson, K., Raub, R.H., Warren, J.A. (1994). Maternal influences on growth and development of full-sibling foals. *J. Anim. Sci.* 72, 1661-1666.

Portus, B.J., Reilas, T., Katila, T. (2005). Effect of seminal plasma on uterine inflammation, contractility and pregnancy rates in mares. *Equine Vet. J.* 37, 100–105.

Proudman, C.J., Holdstock, N.B. (2000) Investigation of an outbreak of tapeworm-associated colic in a training yard. *Equine Vet. J. Suppl.* (32), 37-41.

Proudman, C.J. (1992). A two year, prospective survey of equine colic in general practice. *Equine Vet. J.* 24(2), 90-93.

Pupkin, M.J., Schomberg, D,W., Nagey, D.A., Crenshaw, C. (1975). Effects of exogenous dehydroepiandrosterone upon feto-placental biosynthesis of estrogens and its effect upon uterine blood flow in the term pregnant ewe. *Am. J. Obstet. Gynecol.* 121, 227–232.

Putney, D.J., Mullins, S., Thatcher, W.W., Drost, M., Gross, T.S. (1989). Embryonic development in superovulated dairy cattle exposed to elevated ambient temperatures between the onset of estrus and insemination. *Anim. Reprod. Sci.* 19, 37-51.

Quinn, B.A., Hayes, M.A., Waelchli, R.O., Kennedy, M.W., Betteridge, K.J. (2007). Changes in major proteins in the embryonic capsule during immobilization (fixation) of the conceptus in the third week of pregnancy in the mare. *Reproduction* 134, 161–170.

Raeside, J.I., Christie, H.L., Renaud, R.L., Waelchli, R.O., Betteridge, K.J. (2004). Estrogen metabolism in the equine conceptus and endometrium during early pregnancy in relation to estrogen concentrations in yolk-sac fluid. *Biol. Reprod.* 71, 1121–1127.

Raeside, J.I., Christie, H.L., Waelchli, R.O., Betteridge, K.J. (2009). Estrogen metabolism by the equine embryo proper during the fourth week of pregnancy. *Soc. Reprod. Fertil.* 1741–7899.

Raeside, J.I., Heather, A.B., Christie, L., Rudolf, A., Waelchli, O., Betteridge, K.J. (2012). Biosynthesis of oestrogen by the early equine embryo proper. *Reprod. Fertil. Dev.* 24(8), 1071-1078.

Rambags, B.P., van Tol, H.T., van den Eng, M.M., Colenbrander, B., Stout, T.A. (2008). Expression of progesterone and oestrogen receptors by early intrauterine equine conceptuses. *Theriogenology* 69(3), 366-375.

Reef, V.B., Vaala, W.E., Worth. L.T., Sertich, P.L. and Spencer, P.A. (1996). Ultrasonographic assessment of fetal well-being during late gestation: development of an equine biophysical profile. *Equine Vet. J.* 28, 200-208.

Renaudin, C.D., Troedsson, M.H.T., Gillis, C.L. (1999,a). Transrectal ultrasonographic evaluation of the normal equine placenta. *Equine Vet. Ed.* 11, 75–6.

Renaudin, C.D., Liu, I.K.M., Troedsson, M.H.T. (1999,b). Transrectal ultrasonographic diagnosis of ascending placentitis in the mare: a report of two cases. *Equine Vet. Ed.* 11(2), 69–74.

Rensis, F.D., Scaramuzzi, R.J. (2003). Heat stress and seasonal effects on reproduction in the dairy cow- a review. *Theriogenology* 60, 1139-1151.

Reusens, B., Remacle, C. (2006). Programming of the endocrine pancreas by the early nutritional environment. *Int. J. Biochem. Cell. Biol.* 38, 913-922.

Riddle, W.T., LeBlanc, M.M., Stromberg, A.J. (2007). Relationships between uterine culture, cytology and pregnancy rates in a Thoroughbred practice. *Theriogenology* 68, 395–402.

Rivera del Alamo, M.M., Reilas, T., Kindahl, H., Katila, T. (2008). Mechanisms behind intrauterine device-induced luteal persistence in mares. *Anim. Reprod. Sci.* 107, 94-106.

Rivera, R.M., Hansen, P.J. (2001). Development of cultured bovine embryos after exposure to high temperatures in the physiological range. *Reproduction* 121, 107-115.

Rivera, R.M., Kelley, K.L., Erdos, G.W., Hansen, P.J. (2003). Alterations in ultrastructural morphology of two-cell bovine embryos produced in vitro and in vivo following a physiologically relevant heat shock. *Biol. Reprod.* 69, 2068-2077.

Roberts, S.J. (1986). Abortion and other gestational diseases in mare. In: *Current Therapy in Theriogenology* (Morrow, D.A. Ed.) W.B. Saunders Company, Philadelphia, pp. 705-710.

Rossdale, P.D., Silver, M. (1982). The concept of readiness for birth. *J. Reprod. Fertil.* 32, 507-510.

Rossdale, P.D., Ousey, J.C., Cottrill, C.M., Chavatte, P., Allen, W.R., McGladdery, A.J.(1991). Effects of placental pathology on maternal plasma progestagen and mammary secretion calcium concentrations and on neonatal adrenocortical function in the horse. *J. Reprod. Fertil. Suppl.* 44, 579-590.

Rossdale, P.D., McGladdery, A.J., Ousey, J.C., Holdstock, N., Grainger, I., Houghton, E. (1992). Increase in plasma progestagen concentrations in the mare after foetal injection with CRH, ACTH or betamethasone in late gestation. *Equine Vet. J.* 24(5), 347-350.

Ryan, D.P., Blakewood, E.G., Lynn, J.W., Munyakazi, L. Godke, R.A. (1992). Effect of heat-stress on bovine embryo development in vitro. *J. Anim. Sci.* 70(11), 3490-3497.

Samper, J.C., Tibary, A. (2006). Disease transmission in horses. *Theriogenology* 66, 551-559.

Samper, J.C. (2009). Uterine edema in the mare. In: *Equine Breeding Management and Artificial Insemination* (Samper, J.C. Ed.), Saunders Elsevier, St Louis, pp. 133–138.

Sanderson, M.W., Allen, W.R. (1987). Reproductive efficiency of Thoroughbred mares in the United Kingdom. *Proc. Bain-Fallon.* Mem. Lect., Sydney, pp. 31-41.

Santschi, E.M., LeBlanc, M.M., Weston, P.G. (1991,a). Progestagen, oestrone sulphate and cortisol concentrations in pregnant mares during medical and surgical disease. *J. Reprod. Fertil. Suppl.* 44, 627–634.

Santschi, E.M., Slone, D.E., Gronwall, R., Juzwiak, J.S., Moll, H.D. (1991,b). Types of colic and frequency of postcolic abortion in pregnant mares: 105 cases (1984–1988). *J. Am. Vet. Med. Assoc.* 199, 374–377.

Scott, B.R., Carwell, A.D.B., Hill, A.R.A., Bondioli, A.K.R., Godke, A.B., Gentry. G.T. (2010). A 117 Serum progesterone concentration and embryo diameter on day 7 post-ovulation in mares. *Reprod. Fertil. Dev.* 23(1), 163-164.

Sebastian, M.M., Bernard, W.V., Riddle, T.W., Latimer, C.R., Fitzgerald, T.D., Harrison, L.R. (2008). Mare reproductive loss syndrome. *Vet Pathol.* 45, 710-722.

Sertich, P.L. (1989). Transcervical embryo transfer in performance mares. *J. Am. Vet. Med. Assoc.* 195, 940-944.

Sertich, P.L., Watson, E.D. (1992). Plasma concentrations of 13,14-dihydro-15- ketoprostaglandin F2 in mares during uterine involution. *J. Am. Vet. Med. Assoc.* 201, 434–437.

Sharma, S., Davies Morel, M.S.G., Dhaliwal, G.S., Dadarwal, D. (2010). The Pattern of embryonic fixation and its relationship to pregnancy loss in Thoroughbred mares *Reprod. Dom. Anim.* 45, 61–67.

Sharp, D.C., Thatcher, M.J., Salute, M.E., Fuchs, A.R. (1997). Relationship between endometrial oxytocin receptors and oxytocin-induced prostaglandin F2 alpha release during the oestrous cycle and early pregnancy in pony mares. *J. Reprod. Fertil.* 109, 137-144.

Sharp, D.C. (2000). The early fetal life of the equine conceptus. *Anim. Reprod. Sci.* 60-61, 679-689.

Silva LA, Ginther OJ. (2006). An early endometrial vascular indicator of completed orientation of the embryo and the role of dorsal endometrial encroachment in mares. *Biol. Reprod.* 74:337-343.

Silva, L.A., Gastal, E.L., Beg, M.A., Ginther, O.J. (2005). Changes in vascular perfusion of the endometrium in association with changes in location of the embryonic vesicle in mares. *Biol. Reprod.* 72, 755-761.

Simpson, K.S., Adams, M.H., Behrendt-Adam, C.Y., Baker, C.B., McDowell, K.J. (1999). Identification and initial characterization of calcyclin and phospholipase A2 in equine conceptuses. *Mol. Reprod. Dev.* 53, 179–187.

Spencer, T.E., Burghart, R.C., Johnson, G.A., Bazer, F.W. (2004). Conceptus signals for establishment and maintenance of pregnancy. *Anim. Reprod. Sci.* 82-83, 537-550.

Squires, E.L., Carnevale, E.M., McCue, P.M., Bruemmer, J.E. (2003). Embryo technologies in the horse. *Theriogenology* 59, 151–170.

Stewart, F., Charleston, B., Crossett, B., Barker, P.J., Allen, W.R. (1995). A novel uterine protein that associates with the embryonic capsule in equids. *J. Reprod. Fertil.* 105, 65-70.

Stout, T.A.E., Lamming, G.E., Allen, W.R. (1999). Oxytocin administration prolongs luteal function in cyclic mares. *J. Reprod. Fertil.* 116, 3115–3320.

Stout, T.A., Allen, W.R. (2001). Role of prostaglandins in intrauterine migration of the equine conceptus. *Reproduction* 121(5), 771-775.

Stout, T.A., Allen, W.R. (2002). Prostaglandin E(2) and F(2 alpha) production by equine conceptuses and concentrations in conceptus fluids and uterine flushings recovered from early pregnant and dioestrous mares. *Reproduction* 123(2), 261-268.

Stout, T.A., Meadows, S., Allen, W.R. (2005). Stage-specific formation of the equine blastocyst capsule is instrumental to hatching and to embryonic survival in vivo. *Anim. Reprod. Sci.* 87, 269–281.

Swanson, P.E., Carroll, S.B., Zhang, X.F., Mackey, M.A. (1995). Spontaneous premature chromosome condensation, micronucleus formation, and non-apoptotic cell death in heated HeLa S3 cells. *Am. J. Pathol.* 146, 963-971.

Swerczek, T.W., Dennis, S.M. (2007,a). Equine herpesvirus infections. In: *Current Therapy in Large Animal Theriogenology* (Youngquist, R.S., Threlfall, W.R., Ed.), St. Louis: Elsevier, pp. 176-180.

Swerczek, T.W., Dennis, S.M. (2007,b). Equine Viral Arteritis. In: *Current Therapy in Large Animal Theriogenology* (Youngquist, R.S., Threlfall, W.R., Ed.), St. Louis: Elsevier, pp. 181-183.

Swerczek, T.W., Dennis, S.M. (2007,c). Fungal abortion. In: *Current Therapy in Large Animal Theriogenology* (Youngquist, R.S., Threlfall, W.R., Ed.), St. Louis: Elsevier, pp. 188-189.

Tamby, J.P., Charpigny, G., Reinaud, P., Martal, J. (1993). Phospholipase A2 activity in endometrium from early pregnant and non-pregnant ewes. *Prostaglandins* 46(5), 407-415.

Thorburn, G.D. (1993). A speculative view of parturition in the mare. *Equine Vet. J.* 14, 41–49.

Tinker, M.K. (1995). A farm-based prospective study for equine colic risk factors and risk associated events. PhD *Thesis*. Blacksburg: Department of Large Animal Clinical Sciences, Virginia Tech.

Tinker, M.K., White, N.A., Lessard, P. (1997). Prospective study of equine colic incidence and mortality. *Equine Vet. J.* 29(6), 448-453.

Tremoleda, J.L., Stout, T.A.E., Lagutina, I., Lazzari, G., Bevers, M., Colenbrander, B., Galli, C. (2003). Effects of in vitro production on horse embryo morphology, cytoskeletal characteristics, and blastocyst capsule formation. *Biol. Reprod.* 69(6), 1895-1906.

Troedsson, M.H.T. (2007). High risk pregnant mare. *Acta Vet. Scand.* 49 (1), 1-8.

Troedsson, M.H.T., Ababneh, M.M., Ohlgren, A.F., Madill, S., Vetscher, N., Gregas, M. (2001). Effect of periovulatory prostaglandin F2a on pregnancy rates and luteal function in the mare. *Theriogenology* 55, 1891–1899.

Van Soom, A., Wydooghe, E., Heras, S., Vandaele, L. (2011). Alternative models for the study of embryo-maternal cross-talk and signaling molecules from fertilisation to implantation. *Reprod. Fertil. Dev.* 23 (8), 3-5.

Vanderwall, D.K., Woods, G.L., Weber, J.A., Lichtenwalner, A.B. (1993). Uterine transport of prostaglandin E(2)-releasing simulated embryonic vesicles in mares. *Theriogenology* 40, 13-20.

Vanderwall, D.K., Woods, G.L., Weber, J.A., Lichtenwalner, A.B. (1994). Corpus luteal function in nonpregnant mares following intrauterine administration of prostaglandin E2 or estradiol-17-beta. *Theriogenology* 42, 1069-1083.

Vanderwall D. K., Silvia W. J. and Fitzgerald B. P. (1998) Concentrations of oxytocin in the intercavernous sinus of mares during luteolysis: temporal relationship with concentrations of 13,14-dihydro- 15-keto-prostaglandin F2α. *J. Reprod. Fertil.* 112, 337-346.

Vanderwall, D.K., Edward, L., Squires, E.L., Steven, P., Brinsko, S.P., Patrick, M., McCue, P.M. (2000). Diagnosis and management of abnormal embryonic development characterized by formation of an embryonic vesicle without an embryo in mares. *J.A.V.M.A.* 217, 58-63.

Vanderwall, D.K., Rasmussen, D.M., Woods, G.L. (2007). Effect of repeated administration of oxytocin during diestrus on duration of function of corpora lutea in mares. *J. Am. Vet. Med. Assoc.* 231, 1864-1867.

Vanderwall, D.K. (2008). Early embryonic loss in the mare. *J. Equine Vet. Sci.* 28, 691-702.

Vogelsang S. G., Bondioli, K.R., Massey, J.M. (1985). Commercial application of equine embryo transfer. *Equine Vet. J. Suppl.* 3, 89-91.

Waclawik, A., Blitek, A., Ziecik, A.J. (2010). Oxytocin and tumor necrosis factor a stimulate expression of prostaglandin E2 synthase and secretion of prostaglandin E2 by luminal epithelial cells of the porcine endometrium during early pregnancy. *Reproduction* 140, 613–622.

Watson, E.D., Sertich, P.L. (1989). Prostaglandin production by horse embryos and the effect of co-culture of embryos with endometrium from pregnant mares. *J. Reprod. Fertil.* 87, 331–336.

Wattegedera, S., Rocchi, M., Sales, J., Howard, C.J., Hope, J.C., Entrican, G. (2008). Antigen-specific peripheral immune responses are unaltered during normal pregnancy in sheep. *J. Reprod. Immunol.* 77, 171–178.

Webel, S.K., Franklin, V., Harland, B., Dziuk, P.J. (1977). Fertility, ovulation and maturation of eggs in mares injected with HCG. *J. Reprod. Fertil.* 51, 337-341.

Weber, J.A., Freeman, D.A., Vanderwall, D.K. & Gordon, L.W. (1991a). Prostaglandin E2 secretion by oviductal transport-stage equine embryos. *Biol. Reprod.* 45(4), 540-543.

Weber, J.A., Freeman, D.A., Vanderwall, D.K., Woods, G.L. (1991b). Prostaglandin E2 hastens oviductal transport of equine embryos. *Biol. Reprod.* 45, 544–546.

Weber, J.A., Woods, G.L., Lichtenwalner, A.B. (1995). Relaxatory effect of prostaglandin E2 on circular smooth muscle isolated from the equine oviductal isthmus. *Biol. Reprod. Monograph* 1, 125–130.

Weber, J.A., Woods, G.L., Aguilar, J.J. (1996). Location of equine oviductal embryos on day 5 post ovulation and oviductal transport time of day 5 embryos autotransferred to the contralateral oviduct. *Theriogenology* 46(8), 1477-1483.

Weems, Y.S., Nett, T.M., Rispoli, L.A., Davis, T.L., Johnson, D.L., Uchima, T., Raney, A., Lennon, E., Pang, J., Harbert, T., Bowers, G., Goto, K., Ong, A., Tsutahara, N., Randel, R.D., Weems, C.W. (2010). Prostaglandin E1 (PGE1), but not prostaglandin E2 (PGE2), alters luteal and endometrial luteinizing hormone (LH) occupied and unoccupied LH receptors and mRNA for LH receptors in ovine luteal tissue to prevent luteolysis. *Prostaglandins Other Lipid Mediat.* 91(1-2), 42-50.

Wettemann R. P., Bazer, F.W. (1985). Influence of environmental temperature on prolificacy of pigs. *J. Reprod. Fertil. Suppl.* 33, 199-208.

White, N.A. (2005). Prevalence, demographics, and risk factors for colic. In: *Procceding of A.A.E.P. Focus on Colic.*

Wijayagunawardane, M.P., Choi, Y.H., Miyamoto, A., Kamishita, H., Fujimoto, S., Takagi, M., Sato, K. (1999). Effect of ovarian steroids and oxytocin on the production of prostaglandin E2, prostaglandin F2alpha and endothelin-1 from cow oviductal epithelial cell monolayers in vitro. *Anim. Reprod. Sci.* 56, 11–17.

Willmann, C., Schuler, G., Hoffmann, B., Parvizi, N., Aurich, C. (2011). Effects of age and altrenogest treatment on conceptus development and secretion of LH, progesterone and eCG in early-pregnant mares. *Theriogenology* 75(3), 421-428.

Wilsher, S., Allen, W.R. (2003). The effects of maternal age and parity on placental and fetal development in the mare. *Equine Vet. J.* 35, 476–483.

Wilsher, S., Gower, S., Allen, W.R. (2011). Immunohistochemical localisation of progesterone and oestrogen receptors at the placental interface in mares during early pregnancy. *Anim. Reprod. Sci.* 129(3-4), 200-208.

Wilsher, S., Gower, S., Allen, W.R. (2013). Persistence of an immunoreactive MUC1 protein at the feto-maternal interface throughout pregnancy in the mare. *Reprod. Fertil. Dev.* 25(5), 753-761.

Wilson, S. J., Marion, R.S., Spain, J.N., Spears, D.E., Keisler, H., Lucy, M.C. (1998). Effect of controlled heat stress on ovarian function in dairy cattle. *J. Dairy Sci.* 81, 2124-2431.

Wilson, M.E., Ford, S.P. (2001). Comparative aspects of placental efficiency. *Reprod. Suppl.* 58, 223-232.

Wooding, F.B.P., Morgan, G., Fowden, A.L., Allen, W.R. (2001). A structural and immunological study of chorionic gonadotrophin production by equine trophoblast girdle and cup cells. *Placenta* 22, 749-767.

Yang, Y.J., Cho, G.J. (2007). Factors Concerning Early Embryonic Death in Thoroughbred Mares in South Korea. *J. Vet. Med. Sci.* 69(8), 787–792.

In: Fetal Development
Editor: Josiah Wilburn

ISBN: 978-1-63117-069-0

Chapter 2

COMPARATIVE ANATOMY, DEVELOPMENT AND FUNCTIONAL SIGNIFICANCE OF THE MAMMALIAN YOLK SAC

M. A. Miglino*[*], *P. O. Favaron and A. M. Mess
Department of Surgery, Faculty of Veterinary Medicine and Animal Science, University of Sao Paulo (FMVZ-USP), Sao Paulo, Brasil

ABSTRACT

The yolk sac is a unique structure of vertebrates that has evolved a remarkable diversity of developmental, structural and functional characteristics. In placental mammals, it complements the chorioallantoic placenta during embryogenesis and is involved in nutrient transfer as well as hematopoiesis and erythropoiesis. The latter functions are maintained in the human, where the yolk sac is a temporary structure that participates only indirectly in fetal nutrition. We review what is known on relevant fetal and maternal influences, referring to the evolutionary history of the yolk sac in vertebrates and providing comparative data that includes species used as animal models for human placentation. Topics include the establishment of a yolk sac or choriovitelline placenta, including yolk sac inversion; synthesis, storage and transport of nutritional substances; cellular differentiation; vascularization; hematopoiesis and erythropoiesis.

---

[*] Corresponding author, Tel/fax: +55 11 3091 7690; e-mail: miglino@usp.br.

In addition, we review recent projects on yolk sac derived stem cells. We show that the yolk sac has maintained essential contributions to pregnancy and that it is sensitive to environmental modifications. This may help better to understand pregnancy-associated problems in the human.

INTRODUCTION

The yolk-sac is a unique extraembryonic membrane that occurs in all vertebrates (Mossman, 1987). It displays a remarkable diversity of developmental, structural and functional characteristics. It enables nutrient transfer to the embryo in oviparous species and contributes to maternal-fetal exchange in viviparous species (Stewart, 1993, 2013; Ferner & Mess, 2011). In placental mammals, it precedes and supports the chorioallantoic placenta during very early gestation (Ferner & Mess, 2011; Sheng & Foley, 2012) and is a primary source for hematopoiesis and erythropoiesis (Baron, 2013). The latter function is maintained in the human, where the yolk sac is a temporary structure that participates indirectly in fetal nutrition (Boyd & Hamilton, 1970). However, since significant differentiation of the fetomaternal blood systems inside the placenta does not occur prior to the 10th week, an essential role of the yolk sac for the uptake of histiotrophe from the endometrial glands is likely even in the human (Burton et al., 2001; Burke et al., 2013). Recent findings from bovine pregnancy suggest that the yolk sac and especially its vasculature is sensitive to environmental factors and that it shows severe alterations when assisted reproductive techniques such as artificial insemination, in vitro fertilization and nuclear transfer or cloning are applied (Alberto et al., 2012). Data suggest that high embryonic mortalities may be associated with difficulties in nutrient transfer (De Souza et al., 2001). However, applications of proteomics to unravel functional relationships between environment, genome and phenotype are underrepresented in placentology (Wilkins et al., 1996, 1997; Anderson & Anderson, 1996; Rice et al., 2006; Robinson et al., 2008). Even besides this, the yolk sac is not well understood (Carter & Mess, in press), in contrast to the chorioallantoic placenta for which considerable progress has been made in regard to the molecular mechanisms of substance transport during mammalian evolution (Carter, 2012). Here we review what is known on the differentiation of the yolk sac and associated fetal and maternal influences. This may contribute to a better understanding of pregnancy and associated conflicts in the human.

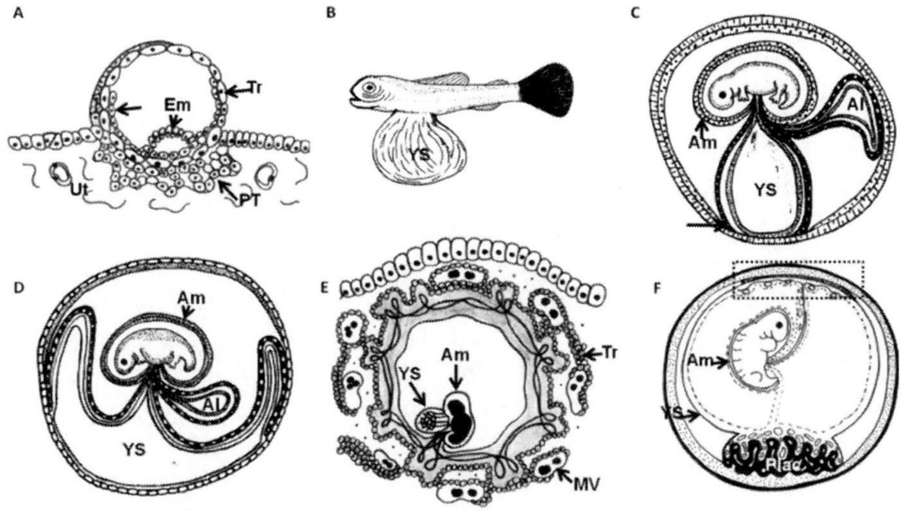

Figure 1. Vertebrate yolk sacs. (A) Blastocyst in a generalized mammal with inner embryoblast (Em) and hypoblast (arrow) that leaded to yolk sac tissues and outer trophoblast (Tr) with invasive areas of proliferative trophoblast (PT) inside the uterus (Ut, adapted after Boyd & Hamilton, 1970). (B) Hatchling of a primarily aquatic vertebrate with persisting yolk sac (YS). (C) Bilaminar and trilaminar (arrow) omphalopleure in a generalized amniote with allantoic (Al) and amnion (Am, adapted after Ferner & Mess, 2012). (D) Invasive yolk sac placenta after rupture of the shell membrane in a marsupial (after Freyer et al., 2003). (E) Free-floating yolk sac without contact to the chorion in early human gestation. Trophoblast of the placenta reached the maternal blood vessels (MV) and substituted their walls (adapted after Boyd & Hamilton, 1970). (F) Incomplete inversion of yolk sac e.g. in the rabbit, in parallel to placenta (Plac) and partly attached to the uterus (square, adapted after Mossman, 1987).

Yolk Sac Developmental during Vertebrate Evolution

A yolk sac is found in all vertebrates and develops by the same principles (Mossman, 1987; Wooding & Flint, 1994): Initially, the yolk sac is formed as an enclosure of the yolk mass by cells originating from the embryonic disc; the enclosed cavity is the yolk sac (Figure 1A). A thin layer of ectoderm, the developing epiblast, forms an outer lining of the blastula as unilaminar omphalopleure. It latter gives rise to the trophoblast of the chorion. The hypoblast (prospective endoderm) then moves inward and develops an inner layer. A double layer or bilaminar omphalopleure is then present. The mesoderm of the primitive embryonic bud, which includes fetal vasculature, migrates between the hypoblast and the epiblast and transforms the yolk sac into a three layered-structure, the trilaminar omphalopleure (Figure 1A). The vascularized parts of the yolk sac are important for substance transfer (Perry, 1981).

In non-amniotes such as cartilaginous fishes, bony fishes and amphibians, the vitelline vessels from the mesoderm transport the content of the yolk sac to the embryo. The yolk sac partly persists after hatching (Figure 1B). In viviparous species, including many cartilaginous fishes, a direct maternal-fetal exchange may occur via the yolk sac. Thus, such species have a placental system build by the bi- or trilaminar omphalopleure. Viviparous species among the bony fishes mostly modify other parts of their body to achieve this end (Perry, 1981; Wourms, 1993).

In amniotes, the situation is different due to the evolutionary novelty of having the chorion, amnion and allantois as additional fetal membranes. Together with the yolk sac, these membranes and the developing embryos are enclosed in the calcified egg shell and reproduction resulted as independent from aquatic environments (Luckett, 1977; Stewart, 1993, 2013; Mess et al., 2003; Ferner & Mess, 2011). During yolk sac development, the expansion of the mesoderm often only reaches the superior portion of the yolk-sac. Thus, both the bilaminar and the trilaminar yolk sac may be present at the same time (Figure 1C). Starting from this basic pattern, a remarkable variety of reproductive traits and fetomaternal associations have been evolved (Ferner & Mess, 2011). Reproduction in sauropsid reptiles varies from oviparity, i.e. embryonic development outside the female body that is entirely supported by the yolk content, to viviparity, where the eggs are retained in the oviduct and nutrients are transferred directly from the mother to the embryo (Shine & Bull, 1979; Blackburn, 1993; Stewart, 1993, 2013; Mess et al., 2003; Bleu et al., 2012; Lorioux et al., 2013). Placental structures are established by the yolk sac or the chorioallantois or both (STewart, 1992, 1993, 2013; Stewart & Thompson, 2000; Thompson & Speake, 2006; Blackburn, 1993, 1998; Blackburn et al., 2010; Blackburn & Flemming, 2012). Molecular evidence has shown a high lipoprotein lipase gene expression in the yolk sac, suggesting that it may be essential for lipid transport in viviparous reptiles (Griffith et al.,, 2013). In oviparous species, the yolk content is the most important source of embryonic nutrition (Blackburn et al., 2003; Almeida-Santos, 2005). For instance in neotropical snakes (*Bothrops jararaca* and *Crotalus durissus*) with seasonal vitellogenesis, the quantity of yolk that can be transferred to the embryo during the first weeks of life is about 2 to 5 % of the total body mass of the newborn. The vitelline vessels migrate to the interior of the abdomen before birth because of a shortening of the vitelline duct (Almeida-Santos, 2005).

In viviparous mammals, a reduction of the yolk content and genomic imprinting evolved (Menkhorst et al., 2009; Renfree et al., 2013). Among them, marsupials are characterized by a short gestation and poorly developed newborn. An egg shell is absent, but the shell membrane persists to near term (Renfree, 1991). A placenta is formed usually by the bilaminar and trilaminar omphalopleure and their apposition to the endometrium after the rupture of the shell membrane, whereas the allantoic membrane usually does not reach the chorion (Renfree, 1980, 1991; Mossman, 1987; Zeller & Freyer, 2001; Freyer et al., 2003; Mess & Ferner, 2010, Figure 1D). Three phases of embryonic nutrition are described in by far the best investigated species, the "grey short-tailed opossum" *Monodelphis domestica*. Firstly, the embryo is nourished by the yolk sac fluid, which receives its content from uterine secretion (histiotroph nutrition). Secondly, when the uterine secretion decreases, the embryo is nourished by nutrients previously stored in the yolk fluid. The rupture of the shell membrane is followed by close contact between the yolk sac to the uterus epithelium and transfer of nutrients from the maternal blood to the embryo (hemotrophic nutrition, Figure 1D). In other marsupials, such as the tammar wallaby, there are only two phases in that access to the maternal blood system is achieved only during birth (Freyer et al., 2003, 2007; Freyer & Renfree, 2009). Choriovitelline placentation in marsupials is achieved in different ways, with the invasive type likely to be the ancestral condition (Mess & Ferner, 2010). Finally, a yolk sac placenta is also formed in many placental mammals. It usually precedes and supports the chorioallantoic placenta during early pregnancy (Enders, 2009). Multiple relationships of maternal and fetal tissues are known (Mossman, 1987; Ferner & Mess, 2011). Data indicate that the ancestral condition includes both the bilaminar and trilaminar omphalopleure as temporary structures, whereas both the early disappearance of the yolk sac and its persistence to near term are derived conditions (Mess & Carter, 2006; Figure 1E,F). However, major parts of the yolk sac are well vascularized by the vitelline vessels and substance transfer is common (Mess & Carter, 2006). A specialized feature among placental mammals is the incomplete or complete inversion of the yolk sac that occurs for instance in rodents and lagomorphs (Luckett, 1985; Mossman, 1987). It is caused by a condensation of the yolk sac by the developing embryo and chorioallantoic placenta (incomplete inversion, see Figures 1F). This condition may lead to complete inversion, where the outer or parietal layer of the yolk sac is developed only for a very short period during ontogeny and then disappears (Oliveira et al., 2012a, see Figure 2A). Thus, the originally inner surface of the yolk sac endoderm becomes close to the uterine lumen and epithelium and facilitates absorption (Mossman, 1987; King & Enders, 1993; Mess & Carter, 2006; Freyer & Renfree, 2009). In addition, the yolk sac endoderm may show phagocytic activity, responsible for ingesting erythrocytes and granules and may act as a region of iron absorption (Welsh & Enders, 1987).

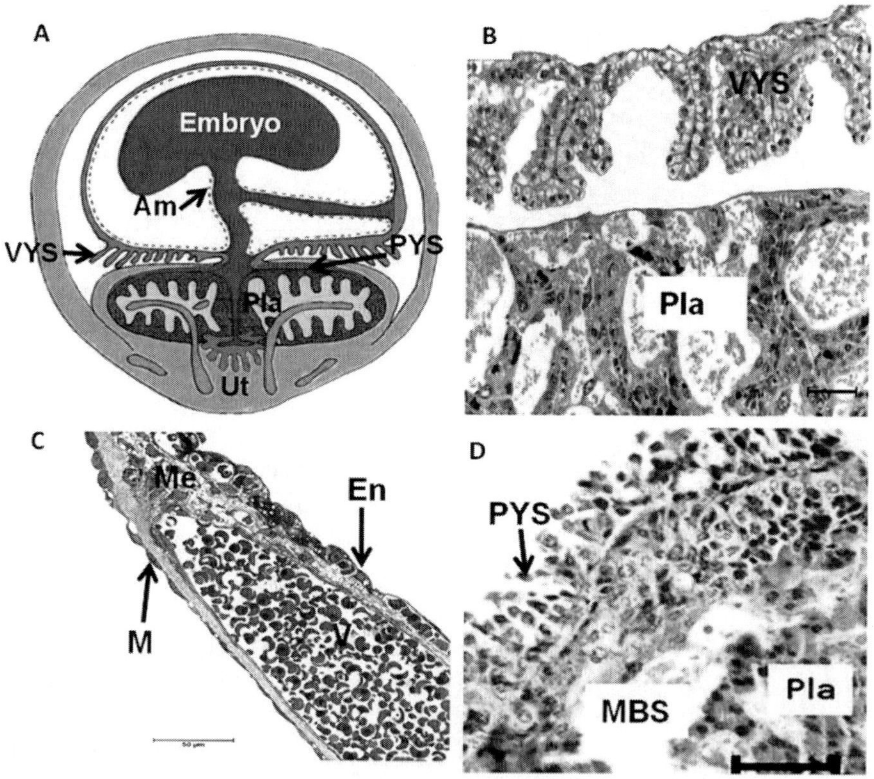

Figure 2. Yolk sacs of rodents. (A) Completely inverted visceral yolk sac (VYS) attached to uterus (Ut) and placental yolk sac (PYS, terminology after Oliveira et al., 2012a) above the placenta (Pla) that both persisted to term (Oliveira et al., 2008). (B) Highly folded villi of the inverted visceral yolk sac in *Necromys*, a New World mice species. (C) Hemopoietic cells in a sac vessel (V) in *Necromys*. En = endoderm; Me = mesoderm; M = mesothelium. (D) Branched placental yolk sac in the guinea pig gestation. MBS = maternal blood space (courtesy B.G. Vasconcelos).

YOLK SAC PLACENTATION IN LAGOMORPHA

As typical for lagomorphs, the rabbit, *Oryctolagus cuniculus,* has incomplete yolk sac inversion (Mossman, 1987, Figure 1F). The ultrastructure of the anti-mesometrial uterine epithelium suggests a very active production and secretion of substances (histiotrophe) to nourish the embryo and fetus. An intense transfer of proteins is reported. Immunoglobulin G is transported into the yolk sac by micropinocytosis (Brambell et al., 1970). The yolk fluid contains all principal proteins of the maternal plasma such as fibrinogen, albumin, α, β and γ globulins in equal proportion and up to 50% of the maternal concentration. Maternal plasma is shown to pass the bilaminar omphalopleure in embryos of the 7th to 8th day (Figure 1F). The blastocyst rapidly expands because of accumulation of the yolk fluid. Later, the inverted yolk-sac, which is connected to the embryonic intestine, acts as an organ of absorption (Brambell et al., 1970; Carter et al., 1971; Mossman, 1987; King & Enders, 1993).

YOLK SAC PLACENTATION IN MYOMORPH RODENTIA

In the mouse, *Mus musculus domesticus* (see Wilson & Reeder 2005 for nomenclature), and rat, *Rattus norvegicus*, the trophoblast and the endoderm of the parietal yolk sac form a transitory area of exchange during early pregnancy that represents a bilaminar yolk sac omphalopleure (Enders & Blankenship, 1999). Later, the parietal yolk sac degenerates and the endoderm of the visceral yolk sac, which is associated with the vitelline vessels of the mesoderm, becomes exposed to the uterine epithelium, resulting in a fully inverted vitelline placenta (Mossman, 1987; Enders & Blankenship, 1999; see Figure 2A-C). The endoderm layer of the yolk sac shows an intense imprinted expression similar to the chorioallantoic placenta, supporting an essential role in fetomaternal exchange (Hudson et al., 2001). Indeed, the cells of the visceral yolk sac have been shown to accumulate and mediate the transfer of proteins by radionuclide-marked retinol (Johansson et al., 1997). Recently, 304 protein spots have been identified to be characteristic for the yolk sac, including proteins involved in nutritional transfer such ad Ash-m, legumain and Cathepsin L. The proteins of the yolk sac are quantitatively and qualitatively different from the embryo proper (Usami et al., 2007). Dunton et al. (1986) used artificially produced giant yolk sacs to study placental transport in the rat. Giant yolk sacs of about 2 cm diameter were formed in cell culture, where the yolk sac cells continued to grow after the embryos died after day 7 (New Copola & Terry, 1973). These yolk sacs were morphologically similar to normal yolk sacs, but the endoderm had greater vacuolar volumes. Close relatives to mice and rats such as hamsters share the same pattern of yolk sac differentiation, but a specialized attachment of the inverted yolk sac to folds of the uterus occurs early in gestation in a New World mouse, *Necromys lasiurus* (Favaron et al., 2012).

Yolk Sac Placentation in Caviomorph Rodentia

Investigated caviomorph rodents include: guinea pig *Cavia porcellus* (Duval, 1892; Demsey, 1953; King & Enders, 1970a; Kaufmann & Davidoff, 1977; Kaufmann, 2004; Carter et al., 1998; Vasconcelos et al., 2013), wild cavy *Galea spixii* (Miglino et al., 2008; Oliveira et al., 2008, 2012a), agouti *Dasyprocta leporina* (Miglino et al., 2008), paca *Cuniculus paca* (Bonatelli et al., 2005; Miglino et al., 2008), rock cavy *Kerodon rupestris* (Oliveira et al., 2006), capybara *Hydrochoeris hydrochaeris* (Kanashiro et al., 2009), degu *Octodon degus* (Mess, 2003, 2007), spiny rat *Thrichomys apereoides laurenteus* (Oliveira et al., 2012b), chinchilla *Chinchilla lanigera* (Tibbitts & Hillemann, 1959), viscacha *Lagostomus maximus* (Flamini et al., 2012), nutria *Myocastor coypus* (Hillemann & Gaynor, 1961), and tree porcupine *Erethizon dorsata* (Perrotta, 1959). The inversion of the yolk sac germ layers is complete from early gestation onward (Figure 2A). However, even for the most inverse pattern, remnants of the parietal layer and original yolk sac cavity have been recently described for a very limited time span during early gestation (Oliveira et al., 2012a). Later, the yolk sac is well vascularized and its villous, visceral endoderm is attached to the uterus and placenta to form extensive surfaces for absorption, whereas the branched placental yolk sac covers the placenta (Figure 2A, D). Distal segments of the visceral yolk sac are non-villous and may be avascular (bilaminar omphalopleure). Recent results indicate that the guinea pig and its relatives are exceptions from the general pattern of placental mammals in that the yolk sac is immature in early pregnancy, but well developed in mid gestation, where it works in concert with the chorioallantoic placenta (Vasconcelos et al., 2013). Intense fetomaternal transfer of proteins and immunoglobulins has been shown experimentally and morphologically

(Leissering & Anderson, 1961; King & Enders, 1970a,b; King, 1977; Kaufmann & Davidoff, 1977; Carter et al., 1998; Miglino et al., 2008; Vasconcelos et al., 2013).

YOLK SAC PLACENTATION IN PERRISODACTYLA

In the horse, *Equus caballus,* the formation of the allantois is delayed and the vitelline placenta is important to nourish the fetus especially in the first 14 weeks of gestation (Perry, 1981; Amoroso, 1961; Steven, 1982; Russe et al., 1992; Allen & Stewart, 2001; Franciolli, 2012). Equines have relatively large, discoidal blastocysts (Mossman, 1987; Betteridge et al., 1982; Betteridge, 2007). A dense, transparent capsule (hard secondary membrane beneath the zona pellucida) produced by the trophoblast occurs when the blastocysts are 3-4 mm in diameter (see Figure 3A) and the developing yolk sac extends mesometrially (Betteridge et al., 1982). Blastocysts of 6 to 8 days show the first development of the endoderm, formed as separate cell colonies sporadically distributed near the trophoblast lining (Enders et al., 1988; Ginther, 1992). Until day 8 of gestation, a consistent layer of endoderm develops from the colonies, followed by a very rapid development of the conceptus (Enders et al., 1988; Ginther, 1992; Betteridge, 2007; Wilsher & Enders, 2012). The horse is characterized by an elongated preimplantation phase with the enlarging blastocyst floating freely within uterine fluids produced by glandular secretion (Enders & Liu, 1991; Wilsher & Enders, 2012). During this phase, the yolk fluid possesses a hypo-osmolality that enables the conceptus to float freely in the uterus, starting around the 10th-11th days of gestation when the conceptus reaches 4-5 mm and maintained until days 18 to 20 when the capsule and spherical format of the conceptus become lost. Comparable environments of phosphate-saline solutions (28 mOsm) are used to maintain the conceptuses *in vitro*. Primary morulas and blastocysts are collected immediately after entering the uterus (6th day) and cryopreserved by standard techniques. However, success is relatively low in horses; especially embryos collected at an age older than the 6th day usually do not survive, probably due to the osmotic response of the blastocyst to the cryopreservative hypertonic agents (Betteridge, 2007; Crews et al., 2007). During early pregnancy, especially between the 11th to 16th days, the uterocalin band of the capsule is involved in the transfer of lipids to the conceptus via the yolk fluid. Additionally, B^{12} micro-globulin is an important protein in this regard. It is not part of the MHC complex class I (heavy α band) as it was not detected in the capsule (Stewart et al., 1995). The yolk fluid contains a low concentration of glucose, but a high one of fructose, proteins, arginine, vasopressin and oxytocin. The concentration of estrogen in the yolk fluid increases continuously for some days until it reaches a plateau. Before the pre-fixation of the yolk fluid takes place, the uterine-globin (p19/uterocalin) easily enters the yolk sac. During fixation, lecithin occurs in the anchorage capsule. At day 21 the capsule disappears because of enzymatic activities and the conceptus becomes fixed and implanted in the implantation chambers of the uterus (Enders & Liu, 1991; Betteridge, 2007). Both the yolk sac and allantois are visible then (Figure 3B) and especially the former becomes vascularized with cuboid, well developed endoderm (Figure 3C, D).

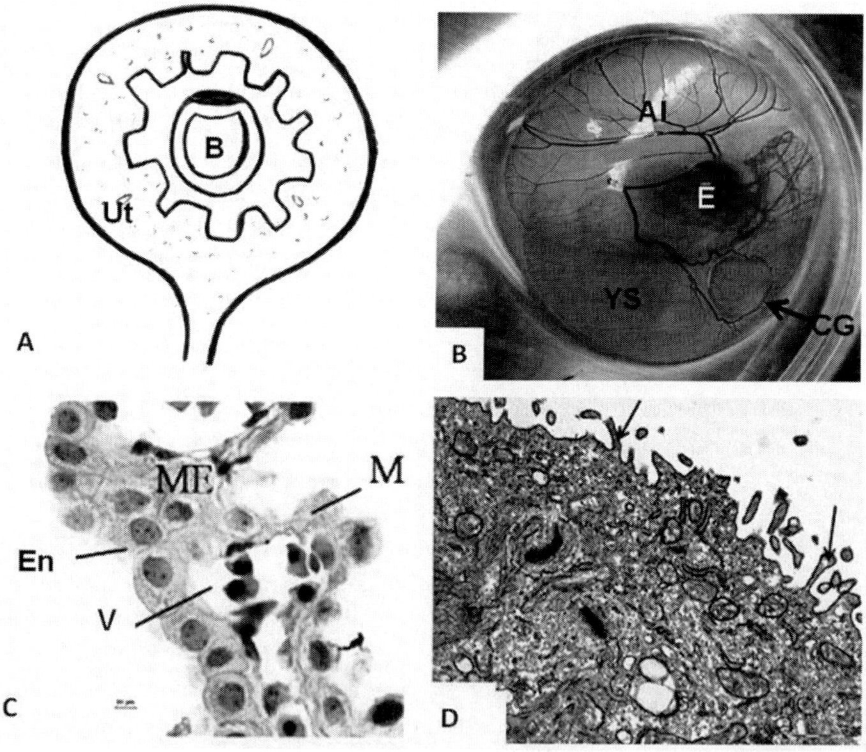

Figure 3. Yolk sac of the horse. (A) Blastocyst (B) with capsule in the uterus (Ut). (B) Early pregnancy with embryo (E), yolk sac (YS) with non-vascularized chorionic girdle (CG) and allantoic (Al). (C) Developing yolk sac vessel (V); En = endoderm; ME = mesoderm; M = mesothelium. (D) Yolk sac endoderm with desmosomes (dotted circle). (B-D: courtesy A.L.R. Franciolli).

YOLK SAC PLACENTATION IN ARTIODACTYLA

In the swine, *Sus scrofa*, the yolk-sac is present only in embryos less than 70 mm in crown-rump-length (Tiedemann & Minuth, 1980). In embryos of 20 mm, the yolk sac endoderm proliferates and forms a simple to stratified columnar epithelium. The endoderm cells show high activities of oxireductases and lysosomatic enzymes, indicating an unspecialized capacity for absorption (Tiedemann & Minuth, 1980). Histiotrophe is secreted by uterine tissues, associated with progesterone and estrogen activity (Roberts et al., 1987). The basal villi of the yolk sac endoderm cells are exposed to capillaries with fenestrated endothelia in the mesoderm. Giant mitochondria with crystalline inclusions are present in the mature endodermic cytoplasm associated with large quantities of rough endoplasmic reticulum (RER) that represents about 60% of the cytoplasm. Most likely, serum protein is produced in the RER and drained to the vascular canals. When the yolk sac is reduced, degenerated materials occur and intercellular and endocytotic canals are frequent (Tiedemann & Minuth, 1980). Explants of yolk sac cells derived from embryos of 30 days have been incubated 3 to 12 hours with [3H]-L-leucine to study the synthesis of proteins experimentally by chromatography, SDS and 2D electrophoresis (Minuth & Tiedemann, 1980). Large parts of the synthesized proteins are bound to the membrane and the albumin (acid protein measuring 80,000 Daltons). Explants derived from the 54th to 57th days have also been incubated. The major radioactive incorporation of proteins then was 69,000 to 70,000 Daltons, indicating serum albumin and phytoprotein. The cytoplasm of the yolk sac endoderm is responsible for the bio-syntheses of some proteins that are shortly stored in the endoplasmic reticulum cisterns. The yolk fluid exclusively contains serum proteins that may be involved in yolk sac regression (Minuth & Tiedmann, 1980).

YOLK SAC PLACENTATION IN CARNIVORA

In the dog, *Canis lupus familaris*, and the cat, *Felis catus*, the yolk sac, which is in inverted "T" shape and closely attached to the umbilical cord, persists throughout pregnancy (Anderson, 1969; Stoffel et al., 1998; Miglino et al., 2006). Early on, the yolk sac membrane is relatively thin with primitive blood vessels, but from day 14 onward the endoderm possesses simple cuboidal epithelium and vitelline vessels are frequent in the mesoderm, forming a well vascularized vitelline placenta (Tiedemann, 1979; Miglino et al., 2006; Aralla et al., 2013, Figure 4A). Small parts of the conceptus are vascularized by these vessels. Detailed, transmission electron microscopy data are available for days 40-60 of gestation in the dog, showing that free ribosomes, mitochondria and rough endoplasmic reticulum are frequent in the endoderm and mesoderm, together with smaller quantities of smooth endoplasmic reticulum and glycogen (Lee et al., 1983). Data indicate a high capacity of protein synthesis in yolk sac tissues (Miglino et al., 2006). In addition, aquaporins have been recorded for the canine yolk sac (Aralla et al., 2012).

YOLK SAC PLACENTATION IN PRIMATES

In a neotropical primate species, the common marmoset *Callithrix jacchus,* the yolk sac develops during early gestation and disappears at approximately 100 days (Hill, 1932; Wynn et al., 1975; Grossrau & Merker, 1984; Bremer et al., 1985; Merker et al. 1987; Enders & Lopata, 1999). In early stages of days 35 to 41, the yolk sac membrane is relatively thin and mainly composed of a simple cuboidal epithelium of the endoderm and some vessels running within the mesothelium (Hill, 1932; Grossrau & Merker, 1984; Enders & Lopata, 1999).

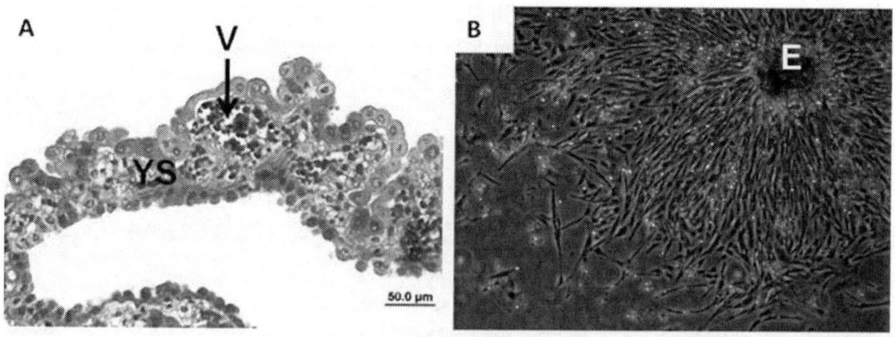

Figure 4. Yolk sac of the dog. (A) Early yolk sac (YS) with developing vessels (V) and blood islands in the mesoderm and simple epithelium of the endoderm (courtesy G. Pignatari). (B) Explant (E) with mesenchymal stem cells from the yolk sac (courtesy P. Fratini).

Later, the endoderm cells increase and a highly prismatic epithelium with prominent folds occurs above the vascularized mesothelium. The endoderm possesses apical endocytic vesicles and microvilli; the cells are interconnected by gap-junctions and desmosomes. Large intercellular spaces occur and the basal membrane is incomplete. The endothelium of the capillaries is porous too. The cytoplasm of the endoderm contains well developed rough endoplasmic reticulum, large Golgi apparatuses and glycogen deposits. Inclusions such as granular secretion, lysosomes and related organelles are frequent (Bremer, et al., 1985). Amino-peptidase M is active in the plasmalemma of the endoderm cells, likewise dipeptilpeptidase IV in the mesothelial cells and alkaline phosphatase in the vessel endothelium. Acid proteases, glucose, non-specific phosphate and non-specific esterase are also produced, indicating that the endoderm epithelium may be involved in the absorption of histiotrophe and lisosomal digestion. Finally, the regression of the yolk sac starts between the 80th to 100th days of gestation, which is relatively late compared to other primates (Bremer et al., 1985).

Finally, in the human (*Homo sapiens*) the yolk sac is of small size, characterized by early degeneration and absence of a connection with the chorion or uterus (Boyd & Hamilton, 1970; Nogales et al., 1993; Freyer & Renfree, 2009, Figure 1E). Besides being important for early hematopoiesis and related processes (see below), recent data show that the yolk sac participates indirectly in nutrient transfer including the uptake of uterine secretion and iron, gas exchange and biosynthesis especially during a critical window between the 4th and 10th week of gestation, i.e. before proper establishment of fetal and maternal vascularization of the chorioallantoic placenta is realized (King & Enders, 1993, Jones & Jauniaux, 1995; Burton et al., 2001, 2002; Jauniaux et al., 2007; Freyer & Renfree, 2009; Burke et al., 2013). The morphology of the endodermal and mesothelial cells clearly suggests absorptive function (King & Enders, 1993; Gulbis et al., 1998). Proteins may be released into the amnion and exocoelomic cavity (Jauniaux et al., 2004). After 9 weeks, the endoderm show signs of degeneration, and increased fibrosis occurs in the mesenchyme (Boyd & Hamilton, 1970; Jones & Jauniaux, 1995). In conclusion, data supports the view that even in the human a form of yolk sac placentation exists during early pregnancy (Freyer & Renfree, 2009).

Hematopoiesis Including Erythropoiesis

Hematopoiesis is the formation of blood cell components; this process includes erythropoiesis, production of red blood cells or erythrocytes, and leukopoiesis that builds lymphocytes, myelocytes and other cells. It has been known since the 1970's that the yolk sac is a primary site for primitive hematopoiesis to produce primitive erythroid and myeloerythroid progenitor cells in the blood islands (Moore & Meatcalf, 1970; Yoshimoto & Yoder, 2009). The onset of definitive hematopoiesis takes place in the fetal liver and placenta, supported by migrating cells, whereas in adults this process occurs in the bone marrow (Baron et al., 2012, 2013; Ciriza et al., 2013). (1) In the mouse, colony-forming (mesodermal) cells are present in yolk sac tissues of day 7 onwards, followed by the occurrence of hemopoietic cells from day 7.5 on (Moore & Metcalf, 1970; Baron, 2003; Ferkowicz & Yoder, 2005; see Figure 2C). In this phase, the mesoderm varies in thickness and possesses cell accumulations that are interconnected by tight junctions and desmosomes and that later transfer into an angioblastic cord (Harr & Ackerman, 1970). On day 8.5 a lumen occurs inside the cord. On day 9, the peripheral cells develop into endothelial cells lining the developing vessels, whereas the central cells lose their cell junctions and turn into primitive erythroid cells or erythroblasts of the blood islands. By day 10, they possess large mitochondria, vesicles and surface invaginations (Harr & Ackerman, 1970). In addition, the yolk sac serves as an autonomous site of B-cell production: the primitive and the definite erythromyeloid progenitor cells initiating from the hemogenic endothelium are present by day 10 (Dzierzak & Speck, 2008; Lux, 2008; Lux et al., 2008; Yoshimoto et al., 2011; Gordon-Keylock et al., 2013). They mainly differentiate into innate type B-1, but not B-2 cells (Yoshimoto et al., 2011). The primitive erythroid cells are present until day 12.5; they dominate the fetal circulation and number several millions. Compared with their adult-type counterparts they are larger and express a unique set of globin genes (Palis et al., 1999, 2010; Fraser et al., 2007). A complex interplay has been reported for the early stages of hematopoietic/endothelial development. After mid gestation these cells are less frequent and their nuclear size and polylysosome numbers decrease and the hemoglobin and cytoplasmic density increases (Harr & Ackerman, 1970), associated with the onset of definitive hematopoiesis in the fetal liver (Sugiyama et al., 2011). (2) In the dog, large vacuoles and dense deposits of glycogen occur in association to erythropoiesis around day 40 to 50 (Lee et al., 1983). However, first endothelial segments occur in the blood islands in association with the formation of blood vessels starting around day 20 to 24 (Miglino et al., 2006, Figure 4A). In the cat, the onset of the primitive erythropoiesis occurs between day 14 to 20 and the definitive erythropiesis takes place around days 17 to 45 (Tiedemann, 1979). Primitive erythroblasts are formed intra-vascularly. They possess polylysosomes, intracytoplasmic, electron lucent channels and nuclear pinocytosis. The dog and cat yolk sac persists after the haematopoietic phase; its endodermal cells, characterized by large cisternae, are an important side for biosynthesis of serum proteins such as albumin and α-fetoprotein (Tiedemann & Minuth, 1980). (4) In the swine, erythropoiesis starts on day 15, when the first blood islands formed by hemocytoblasts occur within the mesenchyme (Sorensen & Hesseldanl, 1976). Hemocytoblasts then migrate to the capillary lumina. (5) In the human, two main processes occur: The initial establishment of blood islands in the yolk sac wall takes place at days 17 to 35, producing a network of vessels lined by endothelial cells with abundant primitive erythroblasts (Baron, 2001; Palis & Yoder, 2001; Pereda & Niimi, 2008; Pereda et al., 2010; Baron et al., 2013). The erythroblasts reach the mesodermal vascular plexuses of the yolk sac and migrate to the liver and other embryonic tissues (Ciriza et al., 2013). Primitive and definitive erythrocytes are present in an endodermal, extra-vascular compartment, the endodermal vesicles, by the end of the 4th week (Pereda & Niimi, 2008). The erythrocytes are pulled out into the yolk sac cavity and reach the primitive gut of the embryo through the vitelline duct, which represents an important, transient pathway for the transport of blood cells before proper vascularization is established (Pereda et al., 2010). The definitive erythrocytes are small, non-nucleated and similar to the adult ones. The extra-vascular localization terminates in the 7th week when definitive erythrocytes occur in the embryonic blood vessels (Pereda & Niimi, 2008; Pereda et al., 2010). Finally, the second wave of erythropoiesis mainly arises from the fetal liver (Pereda et al., 2010).

Hematopoietic and Other Stem Cells in Yolk Sac Tissues

Hematopoiesis requires hematopoietic stem cells (HSC) that have the potential for self-renewal and to differentiate into hematopoietic cells forming the cellular components of blood. They are principally derived from the mesoderm germ cell layer, but usually develop from early aortic endothelium known as hemogenic endothelial cells (Yoshimoto & Yoder, 2009; Eilken et al., 2009; Lancrin et al., 2009; Bertrand et al., 2010; Kissa & Herbomel, 2010). Regulation, self-renewal and differentiation into various cell lineages is controlled by intrinsic factors such as autonomous gene expression (e.g., soluble growth factors) and signaling pathways such as Notch, Wnt and Hedgehog as well as extrinsic factors derived from niche cells surrounding stem cell agglomerations and forming specific niches (Fraser & Baron, 2009; Cherdan & Bhatia, 2010; Sugiyama et al., 2011). Since the yolk sac is a primary site for hematopoiesis, investigations on HSC biology are in focus. Data are mainly derived from the mouse and the human (Auerbach et al., 1996; Yoder, 2002; Chen, 2011; Sugiyama et al., 2011; Moerkamp et al., 2013), but in recent years promising studies have been done on yolk sac stem cells in other animals (e.g., Wenceslau et al., 2011; Figure 4B). (1) In the mouse, cell lineages from yolk sac cell precursors of the splanchnopleura are potential sources for hematopoietic stem cells when isolated in association with the onset of the fetal vascularization and blood cell development (Cumano & Godim, 2001; Yoder, 2002). Such cells generate multiple progenitor lineages that mostly provide short-term myeloid reconstitution in the cell culture, in contrast to cells isolated from intraembryonic tissues that establish long-term lineages (Cumano & Godim, 2001; Cumano et al., 2001). Avarez-Silva et al., (2003) studied mouse cell lineages from days 8 to 17. In phase E8, the placenta, yolk-sac and embryo are not able to produce progenitor cell lineages for hematopoieses. Progenitor cells are derived from stage E8.5 on, first from the yolk sac and then from the embryo. The hematopoietic stem cells of the yolk sac (YS-HSCs) undergo progressive developmental steps when differentiating into specific cell lineages (Avarez-Silva et al., 2003). However, the extra-embryonic YS-HSCs differ from the perinatal or adult HSCs in that they possess greater proliferation activities and different histocompatibility of main antigen complexes. They could be identified by the adult immunologic system even when introduced in small numbers of less than 100 cells per animal (Auerbach et al., 1996). The experimental introduction of new genes to the expanding YS-HSCs via transfusion "*in vitro*" shows that hemopoietic restitution is possible through histocompatibility barriers, resulting as a potential carrier for genetic transfer (Auerbach et al., 1996). (2) It has also been shown for the human that both the mesodermic precursor cells of the yolk sac and the embryo are likewise potential sources for hematopoietic stem cells (Yoder, 2002; Oberlin et al., 2010; Tavian et al., 2010; Ivanovs et al., 2011).

YOLK SAC DERIVED STEM CELLS IN REGENERATIVE MEDICINE

Since the precursors of blood cellular components initially start from the yolk sac tissues, it is hypothesized that pluripotent stem cells isolated from these tissues before the formation of blood islet formation, i.e. on day 7 in mice and day 10 in humans, may originate white and red blood cells, veins, arteries and capillaries (Metcalf, 2007; Medvinsky et al., 2008; Dzierzak & Medvinsky, 2008, Wang et al., 2008). Even though such precursor cells are not fully totipotent, the yolk sac cells are capable of rapid proliferation and are pluripotent in regard to the differentiation into lymphocytes, granulocytes, monocytes, erythrocytes and megakaryocytes (Ikuta et al., 1992; Pallis & Yoder, 2001, Zhang et al., 2003). Such cell lineages do not express specific surface markers or MHC (Major Histocompatibility Complex) responsible for the rejection of tissues; thus, they are not destroyed by immunologic responses and may serve as potential and valuable donor cells for halogenic and xerogenic receptors and transplant experiments (Eskola, 1977). This is a benefit when compared to (1) totipotent cells derived from the blastula and morula, i.e. embryonic stem cells, which may cause tumors if transplanted to adults as well as (2) differentiated mature cells that may be rejected because of histo-incompatibility between the donor and the recipient. Consequently, extraembryonic HSC derived from the yolk sac are a valuable source of stem cells to support existing transplantation therapies in clinical regenerative medicine (e.g., Wilpshaar et al., 2002; Sugiyama et al., 2011; Olivier et al., 2012). Increased understanding of yolk sac HSC biology is essential to improve cell therapies in regenerative medicine and veterinary medicine (e.g. Peters et al., 2010).

CONCLUSION

Since the yolk sac is only temporarily developed in the human, its importance for proper establishment of gestation has often been overlooked. However, available data clearly show that it is a structurally and functionally a diverse system that has an active and complex role in endoderm-mediated substance transfer. In addition, the yolk sac makes essential contributions to protein biosynthesis as well as hematopoiesis and erythropoiesis in vertebrates including the human. Besides this, the yolk sac is remarkably sensitive to environmental modifications such as the application of assisted reproductive techniques. The later methods particularly cause severe alterations in regard to the yolk sac vasculature and blood cell component development. In order to better understand developmental disturbances, ongoing research should focus on in-depth analyses of the ultrastructural and molecular transport processes as well as associated gene expression patterns and quantitative proteomics in laboratory and farm animals. Finally, the yolk sac system provides valuable sources of various stem cells with multi- or pluripotent differentiation potential, but without expression of specific (MHC) surface markers that would cause rejection of tissues or tumor genesis in the recipient. Thus, comprehensive approaches to yolk sac form and function may help to overcome pregnancy-associated complications in the human.

ACKNOWLEDGMENTS

We are grateful to Anthony M. Carter for comments on a former version of the manuscript and help with the English. We thank Paula Fratini. Andre L.R. Franicolli, Graciella C. Pignatari and Bruno G. Vasconcelos for supplying photo material. The study was supported by FAPESP (08/58811-6, 2011/10714-5, 2012/51864-2) and CAPES (BEX0008/13-3).

REFERENCES

Alberto, ML; Meirelles, FV; Perecin, F; Ambrósio, CE; Favaron, PO; Franciolli, AL; Mess, AM; Dos Santos, JM; Rici, RE; Bertolini, M; Miglino, MA. Development of bovine embryos derived from reproductive techniques. *Reproductive Fertility and Development*, 2013; 25: 907-917.

Allen, WR; Stewart, F. Equine placentation. Review. *Reproductive Fertility and Development*, 2001; 13: 623-634.

Almeida-Santos, SM. Modelos reprodutivos em serpentes: estocagem de esperma e placentação em *Crotalus durissus* e *Bothrops jararaca* (Serpentes: Viperidae) [Reproductive patterns: sperm storage and placentation in Crotalus durissus and Bothrops jararaca (Serpentes: Viperidae)]. 2005. Ph.D. Thesis, University of São Paulo, Brazil.

Alvarez-Silva, M; Belo-Diabangouaya, P; Salaün, J; Dieterlen-Lièvre, F. Mouse placenta is a major hematopoietic organ. *Development*, 2003; 130: 5437-44.

Amoroso, EC. Histology of the placenta. *British Medical Bulletin*, 1961; 17: 81-90.

Anderson, JW. Ultrastructure of the placenta and fetal membranes of the dog. I-The placental labyrinth. *The Anatomical Record*, 1969; 165: 15-36.

Anderson, NG; Anderson, NL. Twenty years of Two-dimensional electrophoresis: past, present and future. *Electrophoresis*, 1996; 17: 443-453.

Aralla, M; Groppetti, D; Caldarini, L; Cremonesi, F; Arrighi, S. Morphological evaluation of the placenta and fetal membranes during canine pregnancy from early implantation to term. *Research in Veterinary Science*, 2013; 95:15-22.

Aralla, M; Mobasheri, A; Groppetti, D; Cremonesi, F; Arrighi, S. Expression of aquaporin water channels in canine fetal adnexa in respect to the regulation of amniotic fluid production and absorption. *Placenta*, 2012; 33: 502-10.

Auerbach, R; Huang, H; Lu, L. Hematopoietic stem cells in the mouse embryonic yolk sac. *Stem Cells*, 1996; 14: 269-280.

Baron, MH. Induction of Embryonic Hematopoietic and Endothelial Stem/Progenitor Cells by Hedgehog-Mediated Signals. *Differentiation*, 2001; 69: 175-185.

Baron, R. General Principles of Bone Biology. In: Favus, MJ; Christakos, S; Goldring, SR; Hendy, GN; Holick, MF; Kaplan, F; Khosla, S; Kleerekoper, M; Langman, CB; Lian, JB. Primer on the Metabolic Bone Diseases and Disorders of Mineral Metabolism. Washington: American Society for Bone and Mineral Research, 2003.

Baron, MH; Isern, J; Fraser, ST. The embryonic origins of erythropoiesis in mammals. *Blood*, 2012; 119: 4828-4837.

Baron, MH; Vacaru, A; Nieves, J. Erythroid development in the mammalian embryo. *Blood Cells, Molecules and Diseases*. 2013. Epub ahead of print.

Bertrand, JY; Chi, NC; Santoso, B; Teng, S; Stainier, DYR; Traver, D. Haematopoietic stem cells derive directly from aortic endothelium during development. *Nature*, 2010; 464: 108-111.

Betteridge, KJ; Eaglesome, MD; Mitchell, D; Flood, PF; Beriault, R. Development of horse embryos up to twenty two days after ovulation: observations on fresh specimens. *Journal of Anatomy*, 1982; 135:191–209.

Betteridge, KJ. Equine embryology: an inventory of unanswered questions. Review. *Theriogenology*, 2007; 68: S9-21.

Bonatelli, M; Carter, AM; Fernandes Machado, MR; De Oliveira, MF; De Lima, MC; Miglino, MA. Placentation in the paca (*Agouti paca* L). *Reproductive Biology and Endocrinology*, 2005; 3:9.

Blackburn, DG. Chorioallantoic placentation in squamate reptiles: structure, function, development, and evolution. *Journal of Experimental Zoology*, 1993; 266: 414–430.

Blackburn, DG. Structure, function, and evolution of the oviducts of squamate reptiles, with special reference to viviparity and placentation. *Journal of Experimental Zoology,* 1998; 282: 560-617.

Blackburn, DG; Gavelis, GS; Anderson, KE; Johnson, AR; Dunlap, KD. Placental specializations of the mountain spiny lizard *Sceloporus jarrovi. Journal of Morphology*, 2010; 271: 1153-75.

Blackburn, DG; Flemming, AF. Invasive implantation and intimate placental associations in a placentotrophic African lizard, *Trachylepis ivensi* (Scincidae). *Journal of Morphology*, 2012; 273: 137-59.

Blackburn, DG; Weaber, KK; Stewart, JR; Thompson, MB. Do pregnant lizards resorb or abort inviable eggs and embryos? Morphological evidence from an Australian skink, *Pseudemoia pagenstecheri. Journal of Morphology*, 2003; 256: 219-34.

Bleu, J; Heulin, B; Haussy, C; Meylan, S; Massot, M. Experimental evidence of early costs of reproduction in conspecific viviparous and oviparous lizards. *Journal of Evolutionay Biology*, 2012; 25: 1264-1274.

Boyd, JD; Hamilton, WJ. The Human Placenta. 8 ed. Cambridge: Heffer; 1970.

Brambell, FWR. The transmission of passive immunity from mother to young. In: Frontiers of Biology. The Netherlands: North-Holland Publising Co; 1970.

Bremer, D; Merker, HJ; Gossrau, R. Ultrastructure and hydrolase cytochemistry of the developing marmoset yolk sac. *Anatomy and Embryology*, 1985; 172:101-13.

Burke, KA; Jauniaux, E; Burton, GJ; Cindrova-Davies, T. Expression and immunolocalisation of the endocytic receptors megalin and cubilin in the human yolk sac and placenta across gestation. *Placenta*, 2013 [Epub ahead of print].

Burton, GJ; Hempstock, J; Jauniaux, E. Nutrition of the human fetus during the first trimester – a review. *Placenta*, 2001; 22: S70–S77.

Burton, GJ; Watson, AL; Hempstock, J; Skepper, JN; Jauniaux, E. Uterine glands provide histiotrophic nutrition for the human fetus during the first trimester of pregnancy. *Journal of Clinical Endocrinology & Metabolism*, 2002; 87: 2954-9.

Carter, AM; Göthlin, J; Olin, T. An angiographic study of the structure and function of the uterine and maternal placental vasculature in the rabbit. *Journal of Reproductive and Fertility*, 1971; 25: 201-10.

Carter, AM; Tanswell, B; Thompson, K; Han, VK. Immunohistochemical identification of epithelial and mesenchymal cell types in the chorioallantoic and yolk sac placentae of the guinea-pig. *Placenta*, 1998; 19: 489-500.

Carter, AM. Evolution of placental function in mammals: the molecular basis of gas and nutrient transfer, hormone secretion, and immune responses. *Physiological Reviews*, 2012; 92: 1543-76.

Carter, AM; Mess, AM. Mammalian placentation: implications for animal models. In: McManus, L.M., Mitchell, R.N. (editors). *Pathobiology of Human Disease: A Dynamic Encyclopedia of Disease Mechanisms*, Elsevier; 2014.

Cerdan, C; Bhatia, M. Novel roles for Notch, Wnt and Hedgehog in hematopoesis derived from human pluripotent stem cells. *International Journal of Developmental Biology*, 2010; 54: 955-63.

Ciriza, J; Thompson, H; Petrosian, R; Manilay, JO; García-Ojeda, ME. The migration of hematopoietic progenitors from the fetal liver to the fetal bone marrow: lessons learned and possible clinical applications. *Experimental Hematology*, 2013; 41: 411-23.

Chen, Y; Yu, M; Dai, X; Zogg, M; Wen, R; Weiler, H; Wang, D. Critical role for Gimap5 in the survival of mouse hematopoietic stem and progenitor cells. *Journal of Experimental Medicine*, 2011; 208: 923-35.

Crews, LJ; Waelchli, RO; Huang, CX; Canny, MJ; McCully, ME; Betteridge, KJ. Electrolyte distribution and yolk sac morphology in frozen hydrated equine conceptuses during the second week of pregnancy. *Reproduction, Fertility and Development*, 2007; 19: 804–814.

Cumano, A., Ferraz, J. C., Klaine, J. C., Di Santo, J. P. and Godin, I. (2001). Intraembryonic, but not yolk sac hematopoietic precursors, isolated before circulation, provide long-term multilineage reconstitution. *Immunity* 15, 477-485.

Cumano, A; Godin, I. Pluripotent hematopoietic stem cell development during embryogenesis. *Current Opinion in Immunology*, 2001; 13:166-71.

De Sousa, PA; King, T; Harkness, L; Young, LE; Walker, SK; Wilmut, I. Evaluation of gestational deficiencies in cloned sheep fetuses and placenta. *Biology of Reproduction*, 2001; 65: 23-30.

Dempsey, EW. Electron microscopy of the visceral yolk-sac epithelium of the guinea pig. *American Journal of Anatomy*, 1953; 93: 331-363.

Dunton, A; Al-Alousi, L; Pratten, MK; Beck, F. The giant yolk sac: a model for studying early placental transport. *Journal of Anatomy*, 1986; 145: 189-206.

Duval, M. Le placenta des rougers. IV. Le placenta Du cochon d'Inde. *Journal of Anatomy and Physiology*, 1892; 28: 58-408.

Dzierzak, E; Medvinsky, A. The discovery of a source of adult hematopoietic cells in the embryo. *Development*, 2008;135: 2343-6.

Dzierzak, E; Speck, NA. Of lineage and legacy: the development of mammalian hematopoietic stem cells. *Nature Immunology*, 2008; 9:129-36.

Eilken, HM; Nishikawa, S; Schroeder, T. Continuous single-cell imaging of blood generation from haemogenic endothelium. *Nature*, 2009; 457: 896-900.

Enders, AC. Reasons for diversity of placental structure. *Placenta*, 2009; 30: S15-8.

Enders, AC; Blankenship, TN. Comparative placental structure. *Advanced Drug Delivery Reviews*, 1999; 38: 3-15.

Enders, AC; Lantz, KC; Liu, IK; Schlafke, S. Loss of polar trophoblast during differentiation of the blastocyst of the horse. *Journal of Reproduction and Fertility*, 1988; 83: 447-60.

Enders, AC; Liu, KM. Lodgement of the equine blastocyst in the uterus from fixation through endometrial cup formation. *Journal of Reproduction and Fertility*, 1991; 44: 427–38.

Enders, AC; Lopata, A. Implantation in the marmoset monkey: Expansion of the early implantation site. *Anatomical Record*, 1999; 256: 279-299.

Eskola, J. Cell transplantation into immunodeficient chicken embryos. Reconstituting capacity of cells from the yolk sac at different stages of development and from the liver, thymus, bursa of Fabricius, spleen and bone marrow of 15-day embryos. *Immunology*, 1977; 32: 467-474.

Favaron, PO; Carter, AM; Mess, AM; de Oliveira, MF; Miglino, MA. An unusual feature of yolk sac placentation in *Necromys lasiurus* (Rodentia, Cricetidae, Sigmodontinae). *Placenta*, 2012; 33: 578 - 580.

Ferkowicz, MJ; Yoder, MC. Blood island formation: longstanding observations and modern interpretations. *Experimental Hematology*, 2005; 33: 1041–47.

Ferner, K; Mess, A. Evolution and development of fetal membranes and placentation in amniote vertebrates. *Respiratory Physiology and Neurobiology*, 2011; 178: 39-50.

Flamini, MA; Portiansky, E; Favaron, PO; Martins, DS; Ambrósio, CE; Mess, A; Miglino, MA; Barbeito, CG. Chorioallantoic and yolk sac placentation in the plains viscacha (*Lagostomus maximus*): A caviomorph rodent with natural polyovulation. *Placenta*, 2011; 32: 963 - 968.

Franciolli, ALR. Medicina veterinária regenerativa: multipotencialidade das células da membrana amniótica e do saco vitelino no modelo equino (*Equus caballus*, Linnaeus, 1758). [Veterinary regenerative medicine: multipotential of the cells amniotic membrane and yolk sac the model horse (*Equus caballus,* Linnaeus, 1758)]. 2012. Ph.D. Thesis, University of São Paulo, Brazil.

Fraser, ST; Baron, MH. Embryonic fates for extraembryonic lineages: new perspectives. *Journal of Cellular Biochemistry*, 2009; 107: 586-591.

Freyer, C; Zeller, U; Renfree, MB. Placental function in two distantly related marsupials. *Placenta*, 2007; 28:249-57.

Freyer, C; Renfree, MB. The mammalian yolk sac placenta. *Journal of Experimental Zoology Part B Molecular and Developmental Evolution*, 2009; 312: 545-54.

Freyer, C; Zeller, U; Renfree, MB. The marsupial placenta: a phylogenetic analysis. *Journal of Experimental Zoology Part A Comparative Experimental Biology*, 2003; 299: 59-77.

Ginther, OJ. Embryology and placentation. In Reproductive Biology of the Mare, 2 ed, Cross Plains: Equiservices; 1992.

Gordon-Keylock, S; Sobiesiak, M; Rybtsov, S; Moore, K; Medvinsky, A. Mouse extra-embryonic arterial vessels harbor precursors capable of maturing into definitive HSCs. *Blood*, 2013. [Epub ahead of print].

Gossrau, R; Merker, HJ. Ultrastructure and enzyme histochemistry of maternal blood vessels in the marmoset placenta. *Histochemical Journal*, 1984; 16: 395-398.

Griffith, OW; Ujvari, B; Belov, K; Thompson, MB. Placental lipoprotein lipase (LPL) gene expression in a placentotrophic lizard, *Pseudemoia entrecasteauxii*. *Journal of Experimental Zoology Part B Molecular and Developmental Evolution*. 2013 [Epub ahead of print].

Gulbis, B; Jauniaux, E; Cotton, F; Stordeur, P. Protein and enzyme patterns in the fluid cavities of the first trimester gestational sac: relevance to the absorptive role of secondary yolk sac. *Molecular Human Reproduction*, 1998; 4: 857-862.

Haar, JL; Ackerman, GA. A phase and electron microscopic study of vasculogenesis and erythropoiesis in the yolk sac of the mouse. *Anatomical Records*, 1970; 170, 199-224.

Hill, JP. The developmental history of the primates. *Philosophical Transactions of the Royal Society B: Biological Sciences*, 1932; 221: 45 - 178.

Hillemann, HH; Gaynor, AI. The definitive architecture of the placentae of nutria, Myocastor coypus (Molina). *American Journal of Anatomy*, 1961; 109: 299–317.

Hudson, QJ; Seidl, CI; Kulinski, TM; Huang, R; Warczok, KE; Bittner, R; Bartolomei, MS; Barlow, DP. Extra-embryonic-specific imprinted expression is restricted to defined lineages in the post-implantation embryo. *Developmental Biology*, 2011; 353: 420-31.

Ikuta, K; Weissman, IL. Evidence that hematopoietic stem cells express mouse c-kit but do not depend on steel factor for their generation. *Proceedings of the National Academy of Sciences*, 1992; 89: 1502-6

Ivanovs, A; Rybtsov, S; Welch, L; Anderson, RA; Turner, ML; Medvinsky, A. Highly potent human hematopoietic stem cells first emerge in the intraembryonic aorta-gonad-mesonephros region. *Journal of Experimental Medicine*. 2011; 208: 2417-27.

Jauniaux, E; Cindrova-Davies, T; Johns, T; Dunster, C; Hempstock, J; Kelly, F; Burton, GJ. Distribution and transfer pathways of antioxidant molecules inside the first trimester human gestational sac. *Journal of Clinical Endocrinology and Metabolism*, 2004; 89: 1452–1458.

Jauniaux, E; Johns, J; Gulbis, B; Spasic-Boskovic, O; Burton, GJ. Transfer of folic acid inside the first trimester gestational sac and the effect of maternal Smoking. *American Journal of Obstetrics and Gynecology*, 2007; 197: 58.e1-58.e6.

Johansson, S; Gustafson, AL; Donovan, M; Romert, A; Eriksson, U; Dencker, L. Retinoid binding proteins in mouse yolk sac and chorio-allantoic placentas. *Anatomy and Embryology*, 1997; 195:483-90.

Jones, CPJ; Jauniaux, E. Ultrastructure of the materno-embryonic interface in the first trimester of pregnancy. *Micron*, 1995; 2: 145-173.

Kanashiro, C; Santos, TC; Miglino, MA; Mess, AM; Carter, AM. Growth and development of the placenta in capybara (*Hydrochaeris hydrochaeris*). Reproductive Biology and Endocrinology, 2009; 7: 57.

Kaufmann, P. Guinea Pig *Cavia porcellus*. In: Benirschke K, editor. Comparative placentation. http://placentation.ucsd.edu/guinea.htm.2004.

Kaufmann, P; Davidoff, M. The guinea-pig placenta. *Advances in Anatomy, Embryology, and Cell Biology*, 1977; 53: 5-91.

King, BF. An electron microscopic study of absorption of peroxidase-conjugated immunoglobulin G by guinea pig visceral yolk sac in vitro. *American Journal of Anatomy*, 1971; 148:447-55.

King, BF; Enders, AC. The fine structure of the guinea pig visceral yolk sac placenta. *American Journal of Anatomy*, 1970a; 127: 394-414.

King, BF; Enders, AC. Protein absorption and transport by the guinea pig visceral yolk sac placenta. *American Journal of Anatomy*, 1970b; 129: 261-88.

King, BF; Enders AC. Comparative development of the mammalian yolk sac. In The human yolk sac and yolk sac tumors. Edited by: Nogales, FF. Berlin: Springer-Verlag; 1993.

Kissa, K; Herbomel, P. Blood stem cells emerge from aortic endothelium by a novel type of cell transition *Nature*, 2010; 464:112-115.

Lancrin, C; Sroczynska, P; Stephenson, C; Allen, T; Kouskoff, V; Lacaud, G. The haemangioblast generates haematopoietic cells through a haemogenic endothelium stage. *Nature*, 2009; 457: 892-5.

Lee, SY; Anderson, JW; Scott GL; Mossman, HW. Ultrastructure of the placenta and fetal membranes of the dog: II. The yolk sac. *American Journal of Anatomy*, 1983; 166: 313-327.

Leissring, JC; Anderson, JW. The transfer of serum proteins from mother to young in the guinea pig. I. Prenatal rates and routes. *American Journal of Anatomy*, 1961; 109: 149-55.

Lorioux, S; Vaugoyeau, M; Denardo, DF; Clobert, J; Guillon, M; Lourdais, O. Stage dependence of phenotypical and phenological maternal effects: insight into squamate reptile reproductive strategies. *American Naturalist*, 2013; 182: 223-33.

Luckett, WP. Superordinal and intraordinal affinities of rodents: developmental evidence from the dentition and placentation. In: Luckett WP, Hartenberger JL, editors. Evolutionary Relationships among rodents. New York: Plenum Press, Nato ASI-Series; 1985.

Lux, CT; Yoshimoto, M; McGrath, K; Conway, SJ; Palis, J; Yoder, MC. All primitive and definitive hematopoietic progenitor cells emerging before

E10 in the mouse embryo are products of the yolk sac. *Blood*, 2008; 111: 3435-8.

Medvinsky, A; Taoudi, S; Mendes, S; Dzierzak, E. Analysis and manipulation of hematopoietic progenitor and stem cells from murine embryonic tissues. *Current Protocols in Stem Cell Biology*, 2008; Chapter 2: Unit 2A.6.

Menkhorst, E; Nation, A; Cui, S; Selwood, L. Evolution of the shell coat and yolk in amniotes: a marsupial perspective. *Journal of Experimental Zoology Part B Molecular and Developmental Evolution*, 2009; 312: 625-38.

Merker, HJ; Bremer, D; Barrach, HJ; Gossrau, R. The basement membrane of the persisting maternal blood vessels in the placenta of *Callithrix jacchus. Anatomy and Embryology*, 1987; 176: 87-97.

Mess, A. Development of the chorioallantoic placenta in *Octodon degus*: a model for growth processes in caviomorph rodents? *Journal of Experimental Zoology Part B Molecular and Developmental Evolution*, 2007; 308: 371-83.

Mess, A. Evolutionary transformations of chorioallantoic placental characters in Rodentia with special reference to hystricognath species. *Journal of Experimental Zoology*, 2003; 299: 78-98.

Mess, A; Blackburn, DG; Zeller, U. Evolutionary transformations of fetal membranes and reproductive strategies. *Journal of Experimental Zoology Part A Comparative Experimental Biology*. 2003; 299(1):3-12.

Mess, A; Carter, AM. Evolutionary transformations of fetal membrane characters in Eutheria with special reference to Afrotheria. *Journal of Experimental Zoology Part B Molecular and Developmental Evolution*, 2006; 306: 140-63.

Mess, AM; Ferner, KJ. Evolution and development of gas exchange structures in Mammalia: the placenta and the lung. *Respiratory Physiology and Neurobiology*, 2010; 173: S74-82.

Metcalf, D. Concise review: hematopoietic stem cells and tissue stem cells: current concepts and unanswered questions. *Stem Cells*, 2007; 25:2390-5.

Miglino, MA; Ambrósio, CE; Martins, DS; Pfarrer, C; Leiser, R. The carnivore pregnancy: the development of the embryo and fetal membranes. *Theriogenology*, 2006; 66: 1699-1702.

Miglino, MA; Franciolli, ALR; de Oliveira, MF; Ambrósio, CE; Bonatelli, M; Fernandes Machado, MR; Mess M. Development of the inverted yolk sac in three species of caviids (Rodentia, Caviomorpha, Caviidae). *Placenta*, 2008; 29: 278-252.

Minuth, WW; Tiedemann, K. The pig yolk sac II. *Histochemistry*, 1980; 68:147-158.

Moerkamp, AT; Paca, A; Goumans, MJ; Kunath, T; Kruithof, BP; Kruithof-de Julio, M. Extraembryonic endoderm cells as a model of endoderm development. *Development, Growth and Differentiation*, 2013; 55: 301-8.

Moore, MAS; Metcalf, D. Ontogeny of the haemotopoietic system: yolk sac origin of in vivo colony forming cells in developing mouse embryo. *British Journal of Haematology*, 1970; 18: 279-296.

Mossman, HW. Vertebrate fetal membranes: comparative ontogeny and morphology; evolution; phylogenetic significance: basic functions; research opportunities. London: The Macmillan Press, 1987.

New, DAT; Coppola, PJ; Terry, S. Culture of explanted rat embryos in rotating tubes. *Journal of Reproduction and Fertility*, 1973; 35: 135-138.

Nogales, FF; Beltran, E; Gonzalez, F. Morphological changes of the secondary human yolk sac in early pregnancy wastage. In Nogales FF (ed.) The Human Yolk Sac and Yolk Sac Tumors. Germany: Springer-Verlag; 1993.

Oberlin, E; Fleury, M; Clay, D; Petit-Cocault, L; Candelier, JJ; Mennesson, B; Jaffredo, T; Souyri, M. VE-cadherin expression allows identification of a new class of hematopoietic stem cells within human embryonic liver. *Blood*, 2010; 116: 4444–4455.

Oliveira, MF; Carter, AM; Bonatelli, M; Ambrósio, CE; Miglino, MA. Placentation in the rock cavy, *Kerodon rupestris* (Wied). *Placenta*, 2006; 27: 87-97.

Oliveira, MF; do Vale, AM; Favaron, PO; Vasconcelos, BG; de Oliveira, GB; Miglino, MA; Mess, A. Development of yolk sac inversion in *Galea spixii* and *Cavia porcellus* (Rodentia, Caviidae). *Placenta*, 2012; 33(10): 878-81.

Oliveira, MF; Favaron, PO; Ambrósio, CE; Miglino, MA; Mess, A. Chorioallantoic and Yolk Sac Placentation in *Thrichomys laurentinus* (Echimyidae) and the Evolution of Hystricognath Rodents. *Journal of Experimental Zoology Part B Molecular and Developmental Evolution*, 2012; 318:13-25.

Oliveira, MF; Mess, A; Ambrósio, CE; Dantas, CAG; Favaron, PO; Miglino, MA. Chorioallantoic placentation in *Galea spixii* (Rodentia, Caviomorpha, Caviidae). *Reproductive Biology and Endocrinology*, 2008; 6:39.

Oliveira, MF; Do Vale, AM; Favaron, PO; Vasconcelos, BG; Oliveira, GB; Miglino, MA; Mess, AM. Dynamics of yolk sac inversion in *Galea spixii* and *Cavia porcellus* (Rodentia, Caviidae). *Placenta*, 2012; 33: 878-881.

Oliveira, MF; Favaron, PO; Ambrósio, CE; Miglino, MA; Mess, A. Chorioallantoic and yolk sac placentation in *Thrichomys laurentinus* (Echimyidae) and the evolution of hystricognath rodents. *Journal of Experimental Zoology Part B Molecular and Developmental Evolution*, 2012; 318: 13-25.

Palis, J; Robertson, S; Kennedy, M; Wall, C; Keller, G. Development of erythroid and myeloid progenitors in the yolk sac and embryo proper of the mouse. *Development*, 1999; 126: 5073-5084.

Palis, J; Yoder, MC. Yolk-sac hematoiesis: the first blood cells of mouse and man. *Experimental Hematology*, 2001; 29: 927-936.

Pereda, J; Monge, JI; Niimi, G. Two different pathways for the transport of primitive and definitive blood cells from the yolk sac to the embryo in humans. *Microscopy Research and Technique*, 2010; 73: 803-809.

Pereda, J; Niimi, G. Embryonic erythropoiesis in human yolk sac: two different compartments for two different processes. *Microscopy Research and Technique*, 2008; 71:856-62.

Perrotta, CA. Fetal membranes of the Canadian porpucine, Erethizon dorsatum. *American Journal of Anatomy*, 1959; 130: 35-59.

Perry, JS. The mammalian fetal membranes. *Journal of Reproduction and Fertility*, 1981; 62: 321-35.

Peters, R; Wolf, MJ; Broek, MVD; Nuvolone, M; Dannenmann, S; Stieger, B; Rapold, R; Konrad, D; Rubin, A; Bertino, JR; Aguzzi, A; Heikenwalder, M; Knuth, AK. Efficient Generation of Multipotent Mesenchymal Stem Cells from Umbilical Cord Blood in Stroma-Free Liquid Culture. *PLoS ONE*, 2010; 5: 15689.

Renfree, MB; Suzuki, S; Kaneko-Ishino, T. The origin and evolution of genomic imprinting and viviparity in mammals. *Philosophical Transactions of the Royal Society B: Biological Sciences*, 2013; 368.

Renfree, MB. Marsupial mammals: enigma variations on a reproductive theme. *Verhandlungen der Deutschen Zoologischen Gesellschaft*, 1991; 84: 153–167.

Renfree, MB. Placental functions and embryonic development in marsupials. In: Schmidt-Nielsen, K; Bolis, L; Taylor, CR; editors. Comparative Physiology: Primitive Mammals. Cambridge: Cambridge University Press; 1980.

Rice, GE; Georgiou HM; Ahmed N; Shi G; Kruppa G Translational proteomics: developing a predictive capacity – a review. *Placenta*, 2006; 27:S76-86.

Roberts, RM; Murray, MK; Burke, MG; Ketcham, CM; Bazer, FW. Hormonal control and function of secretory proteins. *Advances in Experimental Medicine and Biology*, 1987; 230: 137-50.

Robinson JM; Ackerman WE; Kniss DA; Takizawa T; Vandré DD. Proteomics of the human placenta: promises and realities. Review. *Placenta*, 2008; 29:135-143.

Rüsse, I; Sinowatz, F; Richter, L; Lehmann, M; Schallenberger, E. The development of the yolk sac in ruminants (sheep and cattle). *Anatomy Histology and Embryology*, 1992; 21: 324-347.

Sheng, G; Foley, AC. Diversification and conservation of the extraembryonic tissues in mediating nutrient uptake during amniote development. *Annals of the New York Academy of Sciences*, 2012; 1271: 97-103.

Shine, R; Bull, JJ. The evolution of live-bearing in lizards and snakes. *American Naturalist*, 1979; 113: 905–922.

Sorensen, VW; Hesseldahl, H. Erythropoiesis in pig yolk sac 15 days after breeding. Proceedings of the Congress of the Nordic Society for Cell Biology, 9th, 1975 (Pub.1976).

Steven, DH. Placentation in the mare. *Journal of Reproduction and Fertility*, 1982; 31: 41-55.

Stewart, F; Charleston, B; Crossett, B; Barker, PJ; Allen, WR. A novel uterine protein that associates with the embryonic capsule in equids. *Journal of Reproduction and Fertility*, 1995; 105: 65-70.

Stewart, JR. Fetal nutrition in lecithotrophic squamate reptiles: toward a comprehensive model for evolution of viviparity and placentation. *Journal of Morphology*, 2013; 274: 824-43.

Stewart, JR. Placental structure and nutritional provision to embryos in predominantly lecithotrophic viviparous reptiles. *American Zoologist*, 1992; 32: 303–312.

Stewart, JR. Yolk sac placentation in reptiles, structural innovation in a fundamental vertebrate fetal nutritional system. *Journal of Experimental Zoology*. 1993; 266: 431–449.

Stewart, JR; Thompson, MB. Evolution of placentation among squamate reptiles: recent research and future directions. *Comparative Biochemistry and Physiology - Part A Molecular & Integrative Physiology of Comparative Biochemistry and Physiology*, 2000; 127: 411–431.

Stoffel, MH; Gille, U; Friess, AE. Scanning electron microscopy of the canine placenta. In: Motta PM. Progress in clinical and biological research: new trends in microanatomy of reproduction. New York: Alan Liss; 1998.

Sugiyama, D; Inoue-Yokoo, T; Fraser, ST; Kulkeaw, K; Mizuochi, C; Horio, Y. Embryonic Regulation of the Mouse Hematopoietic Niche. *Scientific World Journal*, 2011; 11: 1770–1780.

Tavian, M; Biasch, K; Sinka, L; Vallet, J; Péault, B. Embryonic origin of human hematopoiesis. *International Journal of Developmental Biology*, 2010; 54: 1061-5.

Tibbits, FD; Hillemann, HH. The development and histology of the chinchilla placenta. *Journal of Morphology*, 1959; 105: 317-366.

Tiedemann, K. The amniotic, allantoic and yolk sac epithelia of the cat: SEM and TEM studies. *Anatomy and Embryology*, 1979; 158: 75-94.

Tiedemann, K; Minuth, WW. Synthesis of serum proteins by the posthaematopoietic feline yolk sac. *Histochemistry*, 1980; 67: 155-167.

Thompson, MB; Speake, BK. A review of the evolution of viviparity in lizards: structure, function and physiology of the placenta. *Journal of Comparative Physiology Part B*, 2006; 176: 179-89.

Usami, M; Mitsunaga, K; Nakazawa, K. Two-dimensional electrophoresis of protein from cultured postimplantation rat embryos for development toxicity studies. *Toxicology in Vitro*, 2007; 21: 521-526.

Vasconcelos, BG; Favaron, PO; Miglino, MA; Mess, AM. Development and morphology of the inverted yolk sac in the guinea pig (*Cavia porcellus*). *Theriogenology*, 2013; 80: 636-641.

Welsh, AO; Enders, AC. Trophoblast-decidual cell interactions and establishment of maternal blood circulation in the parietal yolk sac placenta of the rat. Anatomical Recordes, 1987; 217: 203-19.

Wenceslau, CV; Miglino, MA; Martins, DS; Ambrósio, CE; Lizier, NF; Pignatari, GC; Kerkis, I. Mesenchymal progenitor cells from canine fetal tissues: yolk sac, liver, and bone marrow. *Tissue Engineering* Part A, 2011; 17: 2165-2176.

Wilkins, MR; Pasquali, C; Appel, RD; Ou, K; Golaz, O; Sanchez, JC; Yan, JX; Gooley, AA; Hughes, E; Humphery-Smith, I; Willians, KL; Hochstrasser, DF. From proteins to proteins to proteomes: large scale protein identification by two-dimensional electrophoresis and amino acid analysis. *Nature Biotechnology*, 1996; 14: 61:65.

Wilkins, MR; Willians, KL; Appel, RD; Hochstrasser, D. Proteome research: new frontiers in functional genomics. Germany: Spring-Verlag, 1997.

Wilpshaar, J; Bhatia, M; Kanhai, HH; Breese, R; Heilman, DK; Johnson, CS; Falkenburg, JH; Srour, EF. Engraftment potential of human fetal hematopoietic cells in NOD/SCID mice is not restricted to mitotically quiescent cells. *Blood*, 2002; 100: 120-7.

Wilsher, S; Allen, WR. Factors influencing placental development and function in the mare. *Equine Veterinary Journal*, 2012; 41:113-9.

Wilson, DE; Reeder, DA. Mammal Species of the World. A Taxonomic and Geographic Reference. 3rd edition. Lewisburg: Johns Hopkins University Press. 2005.

Wooding, FBP; Flint, APF. Placentation. In: Wooding, Flint, G.E. (Eds.), Marshalls Physiology of reproduction, III part 1, 4th edn. London: Chapman and Hall; 1994.

Wourms, JP. Maximization of evolutionary trends for placental viviparity in the spadenose shark, *Scoliodon laticaudus. Environmental Biology of Fishes*, 1993; 38: 269-294.

Wynn, RM; Richards, SC; Harris, JA. Electron microscopy of the placenta and related structures of the marmoset. *American Journal of Obstetrics and Gynecology*, 1975; 122: 60-69.

Yoder, MC. Embryonic hematopoiesis in mice and humans. *Acta Paediatrica*, 2002; 91: 5-8.

Yoshimoto, M; Montecino-Rodriguez, E; Ferkowicz, MJ; Porayette, P; Shelley, WC; Conway, SJ; Dorshkind, K; Yoder, MC. Embryonic day 9 yolk sac and intra-embryonic hemogenic endothelium independently generate a B-1 and marginal zone progenitor lacking B-2 potential. *Proceedings of the National Academy of Sciences*, 2011; 108, 1468-1473.

Yoshimoto, M; Yoder, MC. Developmental Biology: Birth of the blood cell. *Nature*, 2009; 457: 801–803.

Zeller, U; Freyer, C. Early ontogeny and placentation of the grey short-tailed opossum, *Monodelphis domestica* (Didelphidae: Marsupialia): Contribution to the reconstruction of the marsupial morphotype. *Journal of Zoological Systematics and Evolutionary Research*, 2001; 39: 137–158.

Zhang, J; Niu, C; Ye, L; Huang, H; He, X; Tong, WG; Ross, J; Haug, J; Johnson, T; Feng, JQ; Harris, S; Wiedemann, LM; Mishina, Y; Li L. Identification of the haematopoietic stem cell niche and control of the niche size. Nature, 2003; 425: 836–841.

In: Fetal Development
Editor: Josiah Wilburn
ISBN: 978-1-63117-069-0

Chapter 3

INFLUENCE OF EXERCISE TRAINING ON e-NOS EXPRESSION, NITRIC OXIDE PRODUCTION AND MITOCHONDRIAL FUNCTION IN THE HUMAN PLACENTA

Robinson Ramírez-Vélez*

Grupo de Investigación en Ciencias Aplicadas al Ejercicio Físico, el Deporte y la Salud (GICAEDS)
Universidad Santo Tomás, Bogotá, D.C, Colombia

ABSTRACT

A regular regimen of weight-bearing exercise throughout pregnancy has been shown to improve placental growth. The goal of this study was to determine the effects of aerobic exercise training during the second half of pregnancy on e-NOS expression, nitric oxide production and mitochondrial function in human placenta. This was a randomized, controlled clinical trial of 20 healthy primigravid women between 16 and 20 weeks' gestation. The pregnant women who were assigned to the exercise group received a supervised aerobic exercise program of 60 min sessions, three times a week. A heavy mitochondrial fraction was isolated from human placental tissue by differential centrifugation. Mitochondrial and cytosol fractions were isolated from human placental tissue by differential centrifugation. A spectrophotometric assay was used to

* Phone: +55(1) 587 8797 ext. 1811, Fax: +55(1) 8578850, E-mail: robin640@hotmail.com

measure NO production in cytosolic samples from placental tissue and Western Blot technique to determine e-NOS expression. Respiratory rates were determined by high resolution respirometry in placenta mitochondria from control and exercised women. Flow cytometry assays were carried out to measure mitochondrial membrane potential and superoxide levels. Combined aerobic and resistance exercise training during pregnancy leads to a 2-fold increase in eNOS expression and 4-fold increase in NO production in placental cytosol ($p=0.05$). Mitochondrial superoxide levels and hydrogen peroxide production rate were decreased by 8% and 37% respectively in the placental mitochondria of exercising women ($p=0.05$). Hydrogen peroxide production and the activity of mitochondrial respiratory complexes were also measured. Mitochondria from exercised women maintained the respiratory function and a good level of polarization. Mitochondrial O_2^- levels and H_2O_2 production rate were decreased by 6% and 26% respectively in placental mitochondria from exercised women. Activity of complex I-III of the mitochondrial respiratory chain was increased by 29% in human placental mitochondria from exercised women. Also, significant increases of 45% and 21% were observed in complexes II-III and in complex IV respectively in placenta mitochondria from exercised women. Moderate exercise can improve mitochondrial function, e-NOS expression and NO production and decrease reactive oxygen species generation at the mitochondrial respiratory chain in human placenta mitochondria.

INTRODUCTION

Pregnancy is a physiological state characterized by hemodynamic changes, such as an increase in heart rate at rest, increased cardiac output and diminished peripheral vascular resistance [1]. These adaptations appear to be mediated to a great extent by an increased endothelium-dependent vasodilation. The endothelial release of nitric oxide (NO) has been proposed as the main factor responsible for the decreased systemic vascular resistance observed during pregnancy [1]. In addition, a decreased production or an increased inactivation of NO has been linked to the endothelial dysfunction that characterizes pre-eclampsia, gestational diabetes and hypertension [2]. Moreover, while pregnancy is referred to as "a state of oxidative stress" [3], certain pathological conditions, such as pre-eclampsia further increase placental oxidative stress and may result in early pregnancy loss, intrauterine growth restriction (IUGR) and impaired placentation [4]. Placental mitochondria are one of the a major source of oxidative stress in pre-eclampsia [3,4]

In recent years, evidence has accumulated to support the popular belief that physical activity is associated with better psychological health during pregnancy [5, 6]. The American College of Obstetricians and Gynecologists (ACOG) [7] recommend regular exercise for pregnant women, including those who are sedentary, for its overall benefits on physical and psychological health.

Physical activity during pregnancy appears to be beneficial to the maternal-foetal unit [8] and may prevent the occurrence of maternal disorders, such as preeclampsia [9], hypertension [10] and gestational diabetes [11]. Other studies have demonstrated that either beginning or continuing regular weight-bearing exercise throughout pregnancy improves placental growth [12, 13]. Bergmann et al., [14] reported that regular weight-bearing forms of exercise influence placental growth and anatomic indices of functional capacity.

Our previous work, showing that 12 weeks of exercise enhances endothelium-dependent brachial artery dilation in pregnant women suggested that exercise-induced increases both blood flow and eNOS expression [15]. The exact mechanism for this remains unclear, but it is proposed that the exercise-induced intermittent fluctuations in substrate and oxygen delivery produce a recurrent stimulus which evokes an overall growth response [8-10].

On the other hand, aerobic exercise enhances mitochondrial biogenesis and performance, favoring tighter coupling between β-oxidation and trichloroacetic acid cycle, and may concomitantly improve mitochondrial function in muscle skeletal [16]. In other tissues, aerobic exercise in non-pregnant women affects mitochondrial function [17, 18]; however, it is not known whether exercise can produce the same effect in human placenta mitochondria. Considering that recent reports suggest exercise may be useful as a therapeutic agent in the treatment or prevention of placental insufficiency, the exact mechanisms by which exercise exerts these influences remain nebulous.

It is currently unknown, however if exercise produces these effects in human placenta. The aim of this study was to determine the effects of exercise training during the second half of pregnancy effect on endothelial NOS expression (eNOS), nitric oxide (NO) production and oxygen metabolism in human placenta.

METHODS

Subjects

Twenty nulliparous women with a gestational age ranging 16–20 weeks of healthy pregnancy and a live fetus at the routine ultrasound scan were included in the study.

Participants were originally deemed eligible for this investigation if they met all of the following criteria in the first trimester of pregnancy: *i)* gravida with singleton and uncomplicated gestation; *ii)* not at high risk for preterm delivery (p.e: alcohol use, drug use, history of smokers, placenta previa, incompetent cervix, polyhydramnios, oligohydramnios, or miscarriage in the last twelve months); *iii)* 18–25 years of age; *iv)* being sedentary before gestation (exercising < 20 min on < 3 days/week); *v)* being under medical follow-up throughout the entire pregnancy period (and planning to give birth) in the same obstetrics hospital department (Red de Salud Ladera, Cali-Colombia); and *vi)* having no absolute or relative contraindication to exercise participation during pregnancy (such as, among others, haemodynamically significant heart disease, restrictive lung disease, pregnancy induced hypertension, severe anaemia, maternal cardiac arrhythmia, chronic bronchitis, type I diabetes or extreme morbid obesity (body mass index ≥40 kg/m^2)). Maternal and fetal characteristics are presented in (Table 1.)

The Ethics Committees of Universidad del Valle and Red de Salud Ladera (Resolution-017/08-UV and SCAH/0408-A/08) approved the trial. All participants will provide written informed consent before entering the study. The protocol was in accordance with the latest revision of the Declaration of Helsinki.

EXPERIMENTAL DESIGN

This study involved a subset of subjects enrolled in a randomized controlled trial to evaluate the effect of regular exercise on maternal endothelium-dependent vasodilatation (A detailed account of the methods used in this study has been published elsewhere [15], from March 2010 to January 2011.

Table 1. Characteristics of the population: maternal age, BMI, gestational age at birth, fetal and placental weight and fetal gender in pregnancies

Characteristics	Control	Exercised
Maternal age (yr)	19.5 ± 3.4	19.2 ± 2.6
Body mass index (BMI)	24.1 ± 4.5	22.9 ± 3.8
Gestational age at birth (yr)	39.8 ± 2.0	38.7 ± 1.0
Fetal weight (g)	3013.2 ± 493.8	3133.3 ± 406.5
Placental weight (g)	430.4 ± 28.9	390.0 ± 20.4
Fetal gender (female/male)	6/4	5/5

Data reported are mean ± SD.

Interventions and Training Program

The pregnant women who were assigned to the exercise group participated in a 60 min supervised aerobic and resistance exercise session, three times a week [15,16]. An average of 32 training sessions per subject was planned for each participant, in consideration that delivery could occur before 40 weeks' gestation. All women had their heart rate monitored during the training sessions to ensure that the exercise was of a moderate-to vigorous intensity. A physiotherapist and a physical educator were present during the exercise sessions. Each session included 30-min of aerobic circuit training accompanied by an audio recording of music and instructions which guided the participants to exercise at each station for approximately 1 min and then move to the next station in three circuits of 10 stations. Participants wore a heart rate monitor (Polar Pacer, USA) in every exercise session which were checked at rest after 15 and 30 mins to ensure that they exercised in the prescribed target heart rate zone. Each session was preceded and followed by a gradual warm-up and cool down period which were both of 10 min duration and consisted of walking and light, static stretching (avoiding muscle pain) of major muscle groups (upper and lower limbs, neck and trunk muscles). The cool down period also included relaxation and stretching exercises.

Resistance exercises were performed through the full range of motion normally associated with correct technique for each exercise and engaged the major muscle groups (abdominal, dorsal, shoulder, upper and lower limb muscles). They included 5 exercise groups circuit training (50 repetitions of each) using barbells (1-3 kg/exercise) or low-to-medium resistance bands

(Therabands). Each type of exercise on the back was performed for 2 min. As a general rule and to reduce potential risks, we excluded activities that promoted that Valsalva maneuver, ballistic or plyometric exercises and positions of extreme muscular tension.

The control group received no intervention; that is, participants neither attended the exercise classes nor took part in an exercise program at home. Both groups continued with their normal prenatal care and physical activity. Each woman met with the study dietician for nutrition assessment and counselling, and an individualized nutrition intervention plan was developed from the baseline food intake assessment, participant preferences, and the meal plan [19, 17]. On a weekly basis, each participant all participants received a light breakfast/meal 45 min before the exercise session which typically consisted of a meal designed to promote weight and recommended during pregnancy (approximately (400 kcal) [carbohydrate to 40–55 %, fat 30 % and 20–30 % to protein of total energy) [20]. The food records were analyzed for nutritional content and caloric intake using the ESHA Food Processor SQL (version 9.8; Canadian Nutrient File database). The participants received support for public transport to attend the exercise classes (US10 per session).

Tissue Preparation and Sampling

Placentas were collected within 15 min of delivery. The maternal decidua was removed and the central portion between the maternal and fetal surfaces used in the preparation. Maternal villous tissue (100 g) was chopped into small pieces, washed with NaCl 0.9 per cent to remove blood and filtered through gauze.

Isolation of Human Placental Mitochondria

Human placental mitochondria were obtained with the modified protocol of differential centrifugation, previously described by Martinez et al., [21, 22]. Briefly, several placental cotyledons were removed from the maternal side of the placenta and placed immediately into an ice-cold medium containing MSHE buffer (210 mM mannitol, 70 mM sucrose, 5 mM Hepes, 1 mM EDTA, pH 7.4). All steps were carried out at 4°C. Soft villous tissue (4-7g) was freed from connective tissue and minced into small pieces with scissors.

The tissue was washed with the same solution and then filtered three times through a thin surgical gauze layer. The tissue was re-suspended in the same medium and homogenized with a Potter-Elvehjem homogenizer (7 up-and-down strokes). The homogenate was centrifuged at 1,500 g for 10 min in a refrigerated centrifuge. The supernatant was recovered and centrifuged at 4,000 g for 15 min to pellet large mitochondria (predominantly cytotrophoblast mitochondria) was resuspended in a minimal volume of respiratory medium containing MSH buffer (210 mM mannitol, 70 mM sucrose, 5 mM Hepes, pH 7.4) adjusted to pH 7.4. A part of the isolated mitochondrial fraction was frozen at -80°C until the enzyme assays were performed. This method has previously been shown to yield mitochondria free from contaminants from other parts of the cell. This method yields a total mitochondrial protein content estimated between 1-2 mg/g of wet placental tissue.

Endothelial NOS Expression

The frozen placental tissue were thawed and minced into small pieces and homogenized in cell lysis buffer containing 100 mM Tris, 50 mM NaCl, 10 mM EDTA, 1% TritonX-100. Insoluble placenta tissues were removed by centrifugation at 3.000 g, 4°C, for 10 min. Samples were loaded and subjected to SDS-PAGE in 7.5% polyacrylamide gels. After electrophoresis, proteins were electro-transferred to nitrocellulose membrane (Amersham Biosciences; Piscataway, NJ). Equal loading of samples (80 μg) and even transfer efficiency were monitored with the use of 0.5% Ponceau S staining of the blot membrane.

The blot membrane was then incubated in a blocking buffer (5% nonfat dry milk, 10 mM Tris-HCl, pH 7.6, 150 mM NaCl, and 0.1% Tween 20) for 2 h at room temperature and then probed with a rabbit polyclonal antibody against the endothelial isoform of NOS (amino terminus, H-299, Santa Cruz Biotechnology, Santa Cruz, CA, USA: dilution 1:500) at room temperature. The nitrocellulose membrane was subsequently incubated with a secondary goat anti-rabbit antibody conjugated with horseradish peroxidase (HRP) (dilution 1:1000), and revealed by chemiluminescence with ECL reagent (Amersham Biosciences; Piscataway, NJ). Densitometric analysis of the eNOS bands was performed using the NIH Image 1.54 software. β-actin expression levels were used to normalize the results [21].

NOS Activity

Nitric oxide production was measured in cytosolic fractions using a spectrophotometric method by following the oxidation of oxyhemoglobin to methemoglobin at 37 °C, in a reaction medium containing 50 mM phosphate buffer (pH 5.8 for mitochondrial preparations and pH 7.4 for the cytosolic fractions), 1 mM $CaCl_2$, 50 μM L-arginine, 100 μM NADPH, 10 μM dithiothreitol (DTT), 4 μM Cu-Zn superoxide dismutase (SOD) (to avoid interference by O_2^-), 0.1 μM catalase (to avoid oxyhemoglobin oxidation by H_2O_2), 0.5–1.0 mg submitochondrial protein/ml and 25 μM oxyhemoglobin (expressed per heme group). Kinetics were followed at 577–591 nm (ε=11.2 mM^{-1} cm^{-1}) in a double-beam double wave length spectrophotometer (Beckman-Coulter Series DU) [23].

Oxygen Metabolism

Superoxide anion (O_2^-) was detected using the fluorogenic dye MitoSOX ($C_{43}H_{34}N_3IP$) a membrane permeant and rapidly targeted mitochondrial O_2^- indicator for living cells, with excitation/emission maxim of 510/580 nm. Based on the ability of the positively charged TPP^+ moiety of MitoSox Red to accumulate in the mitochondrial matrix, and also due to its ability to intercalate into mtDNA, a sufficient amount of this probe is retained in the matrix. Both MitoSox Red free and DNA-intercalated forms are sensitive to O_2^-. We developed a special protocol by flow cytometry in order to detect superoxide anion not consumed by the MnSOD in isolated mitochondria. Isolated mitochondria from placental tissue were loaded with 2.5 μM MitoSOX, during 20 min at 37ºC, in the same MSH buffer supplemented with malate plus glutamate. Antimycin A (0.5 μM), an inhibitor of the ubiquinone–cytochrome c reductase, was used as a positive control. Auto fluorescence was evaluated in samples without probe. Hydrogen peroxide (H_2O_2) generation was determined in intact isolated human placental mitochondria by the scopoletin-HRP method following the decrease in fluorescence intensity at 365-450 nm (λ exc-λ em) at 37°C [24]. The reaction medium consisted of 0.23 M mannitol, 0.07 M sucrose, 20 mM Tris-HCl (pH 7.4), 0.8 μM HRP, 1 μM scopoletin, 0.3 μM SOD to ensure that all O_2^- was converted to H_2O_2; 6 mM succinate plus glutamate were used as substrates. Calibration was made using H_2O_2 (0.05-0.35 μM) as standard to express the fluorescence changes as nmol

H_2O_2/min.mg protein. H_2O_2 production was highly sensitive to catalase addition (3.500 U/ml).

Mitochondrial Respiratory Function

The oxygen consumption in isolated human placental mitochondria was assayed with a high-resolution respirometry (Oroboros Oxygraph, Paar KG, Graz, Austria). Mitochondrial protein (0.5 –1mg/ml) in a reaction medium consisting of 0.23 M mannitol, 0.07 M sucrose, 20 mM Tris-HCl, 5 mM malate plus glutamate, 5 mM PO4H2K, 4 mM $MgCl_2$ (pH 7.4), and 0.2% bovine serum albumin, at 30° C was used. State 3 was estimated by the addition of 1 mM ADP and the respiratory control ratio was calculated from the ratio of the state 3/state 4 respiratory rates with and without ADP, respectively [25].

Mitochondrial Respiratory Complexes I-IV

NADH-cytochrome c reductase activity (complex I-III) was measured in isolated human placental mitochondria from control and exercise women by following spectrophotometrically the reduction of cytochrome c at 550 nm (λ=19.6 mM-1cm-1) in a reaction medium containing 100 mM phosphate buffer (pH 7.4), 0.2 mM NADH, 0.1 mM cytochrome c and 0.5 mM KCN at 30°C. Enzyme activity was expressed in nmoles cytochrome c reduced per minute per mg of protein. Succinate cytochrome c reductase activity (complex II+III) was similarly determined and expressed, except that NADH was substituted by 20 mM succinate. Cytochrome oxidase activity (complex IV) was assayed spectrophotometrically at 550 nm by following the rate of oxidation of 50 μM ferrocytochrome c [26]. The activity was expressed as nmoles cytochrome c oxidized per minute per mg of protein.

Maternal and Conceptus Morphometrics

Study investigators were informed when any study participant was admitted for delivery, and were present to monitor labor and delivery and to collect data. Gestational age at the time of delivery (in weeks and days) was recorded from hospital perinatal records. Anthropometric measurements of newborns: birth weight and placental weight (SECA scale ± 10 g), were taken one hour after delivery by standard methods [13,14]. Placental efficiency was defined as the fetal weight/placental weight, as described previously [13,14]

Protein Assays

Determination of mitochondrial protein was determined by the Lowry assay [27] using bovine serum albumin as the standard (Bio-Rad Protein Assay). All experiments were performed in triplicate.

Statistical Analysis

All the data were subjected to statistical analyses using the SAS program. Maternal and fetal characteristics presented were expressed as means ± SE. Values in figures are the mean ± SEM. Statistical comparisons of superoxide anion level and NO production by groups were performed with two-way ANOVA. Intra-patient comparisons are tested with Mann-Whitney's U test. The eNOS activity, H_2O production, placental weight and placental efficiency were compared by Mann-Whitney's U test. A difference was considered to be statistically significant when $p<0.05$.

RESULTS

Compliance with the Trial Method

From enrollment to at least 28-32 wk gestation, the mean participation of the active subjects was 28.9 out of 36 (SD 3.2) sessions over the 12 weeks. No participant experienced adverse events during or after the exercise.

eNOS Expression and NO Production

Figure 1 shows that in pregnant women 12 weeks of exercise training resulted in a 4-fold increase in eNOS/β-actin expression in cytosolic samples (p<0.05). A 2-fold increase in NO production was also observed in their cytosolic samples (p<0.05) (Figure 2).

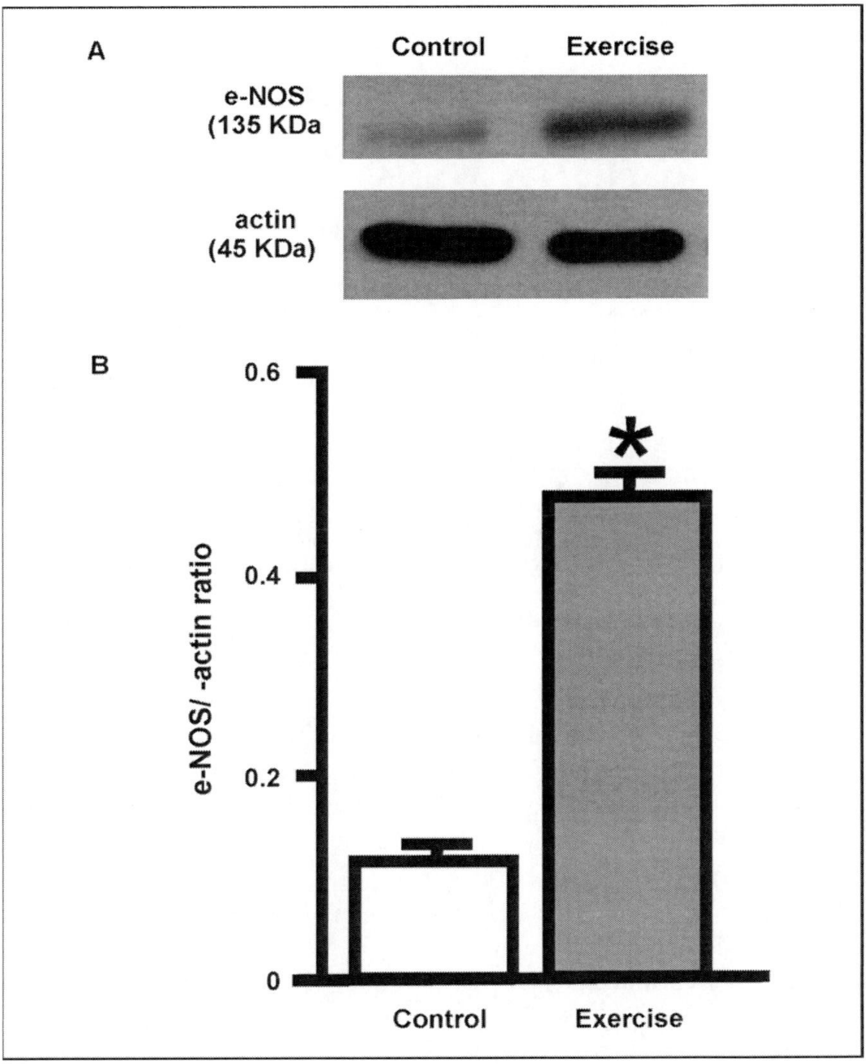

Figure 1. Effects of physical exercise on eNOS protein expression. (A) Typical examples of Western blots for placental cytosolic fractions for each experimental group. Each blot was normalized to expression of β-actin from the same gel. (B) Bars represent cytosolic eNOS/β-actin ratios ± SEM obtained after densitometric analysis. (*$p < 0.05$, as compared with control value). The results shown are representative of three independent studies.

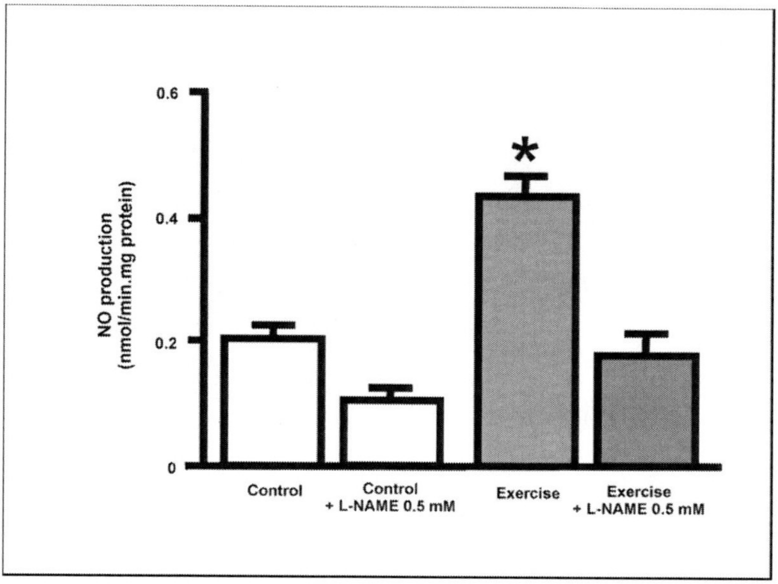

Figure 2. Effects of physical exercise on NO production in cytosolic samples from placental tissue. The specificity of the assay was evaluated using 0.5 mM L-NAME. Data are expressed as mean ± SEM. (*$p < 0.05$, as compared with control value).

Oxygen Metabolism

Within the mitochondria, the electron transport chain is the main source of reactive oxygen species, O_2^- being the primary molecule generated by the mitochondrial respiratory chain. The mitochondria were loaded with MitoSOX, a fluorescence probe that typically increases its emission in the presence of an excessive generation of O_2^- escaping from the action of the MnSOD. Quantification of the superoxide anion levels as percentage values of MitoSox r. f. i is shown in Figure 3. Mitosox fluorescence intensity was 8% lower in exercised mitochondria than in control samples. As expected, both mitochondrial samples exposed to antimycin showed higher FL-2 fluorescence values as compared with basal levels.

H_2O_2 Production

H_2O_2 production was measured in intact isolated human placental mitochondria from control and exercised women, using succinate-glutamate as mitochondrial substrates. Hydrogen peroxide rates obtained from human placenta mitochondria were within the range of H_2O_2 production rates previously observed in our laboratory for other tissues e.g. rodent heart, liver and brain [19, 28].

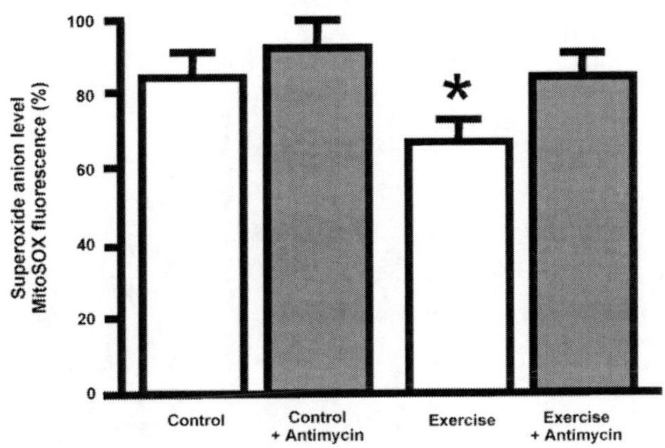

Figure 3. Determination of superoxide anion level. Mitochondrial samples were loaded with the superoxide anion sensor MitoSox during 20 min at 37°C. Antimycin A (0.5 μM) was used as a positive control. Bar graph quantification of Mitosox fluorescence expressed as percentage values of human placental mitochondria from control and exercised women. Antimycin effect is also shown for both samples. Data are expressed as mean ± SEM, from three independent experiments. (*$p < 0.05$, as compared with control value).

Mitochondrial H_2O_2 production rate was approximately 0.51 ± 0.06 nmol/min.mg protein for placental mitochondria isolated from the control women. A 37% decrease of H_2O_2 production rate was observed in the placental mitochondria of exercised women, compared with control subjects ($p<0.05$) (Figure 4).

Mitochondrial Respiration

Malate-glutamate-dependent oxygen consumption rate was measured in state 4 (resting or controlled respiration) and in state 3 (active respiration, with maximal physiological rate of O_2 uptake and ATP synthesis) and the respiratory control ratios were calculated.

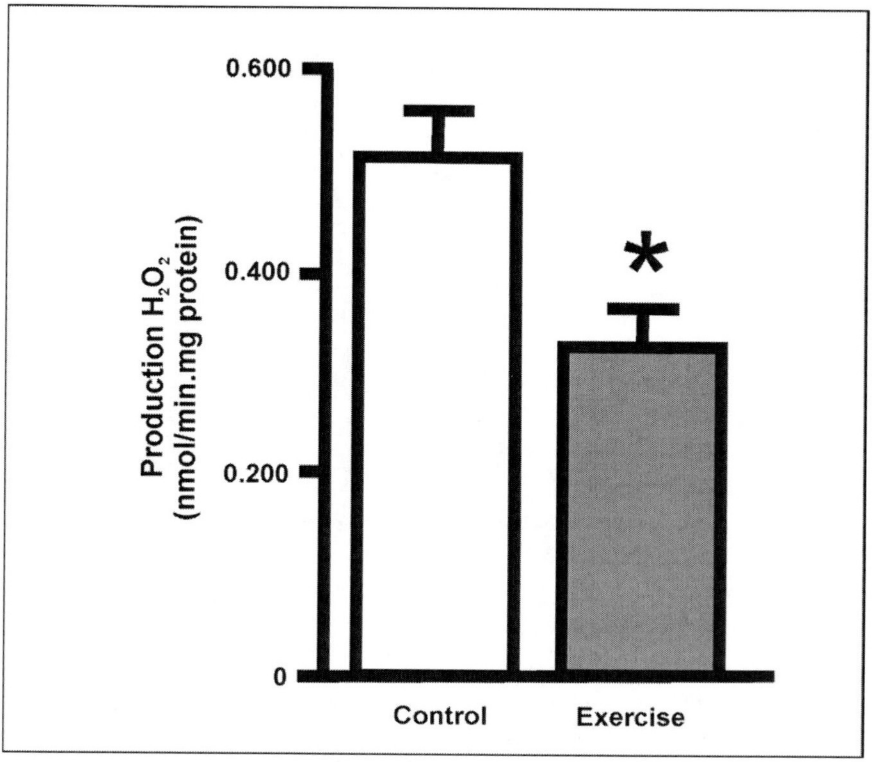

Figure 4. Bar scheme of H_2O_2 production rate of human placental mitochondria from exercised or control subjects. Data are expressed as mean ± SEM of 4-6 mitochondrial samples for each condition. (*$p < 0.05$, as compared with control value).

Results are shown in (Figure 5). Human placental mitochondria present a high metabolic activity as indicated by the measured rates of oxygen uptake in the presence of malate/glutamate and ADP. They exhibited respiratory control ratios of 3.0-4.0, similar to those reported by Martinez et al., [21, 22], indicating the presence of a well-preserved inner mitochondrial membrane (Figure 5A). Placental mitochondria from exercised women showed significant decreases of 37% (Figure 5B) and 44% in state 3 respiratory rate and respiratory control respectively, as compared with placental mitochondria from control women (Figure 5C).

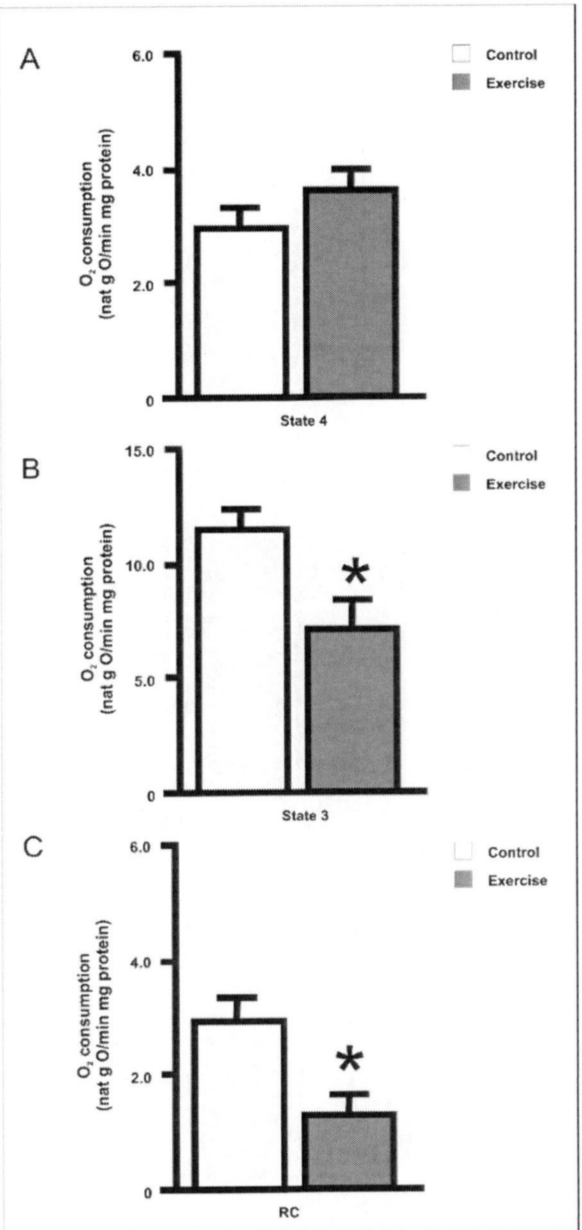

Figure 5. Bar scheme of oxygen consumption by human placental mitochondria from control and exercised subjects. Data are expressed as mean ± SEM of 4-6 mitochondrial samples for each condition.

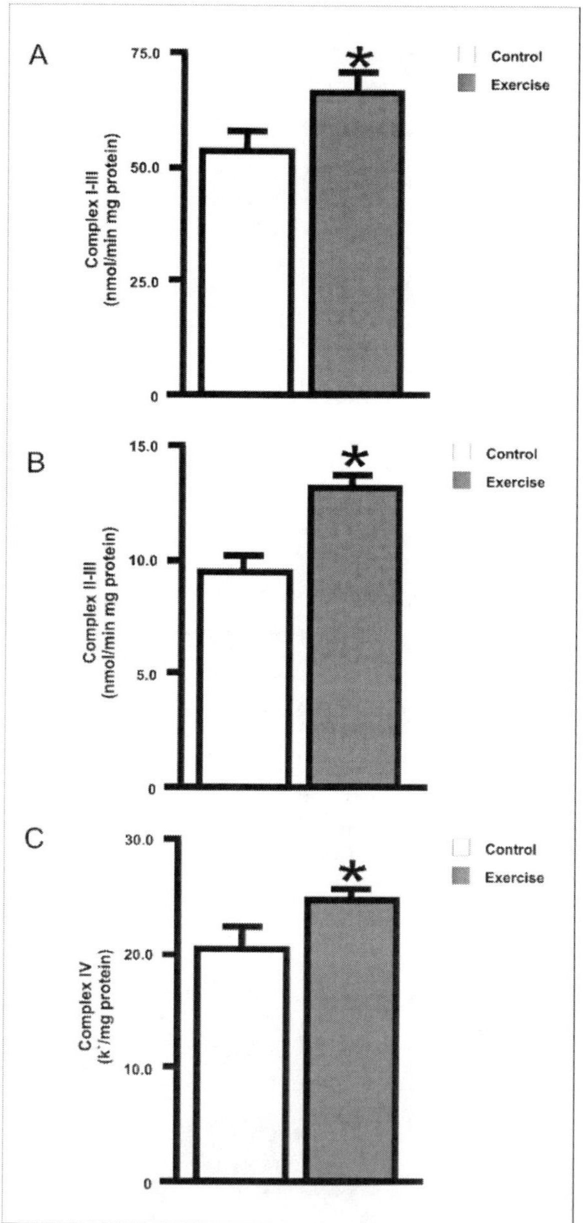

Figure 6. Bar scheme of activity of enzymatic complexes of mitochondrial respiratory chain in human placenta mitochondria from control and exercised subjects. Data are expressed as mean ± SEM of 4-6 mitochondrial samples for each condition. (*$p < 0.05$, as compared with control value).

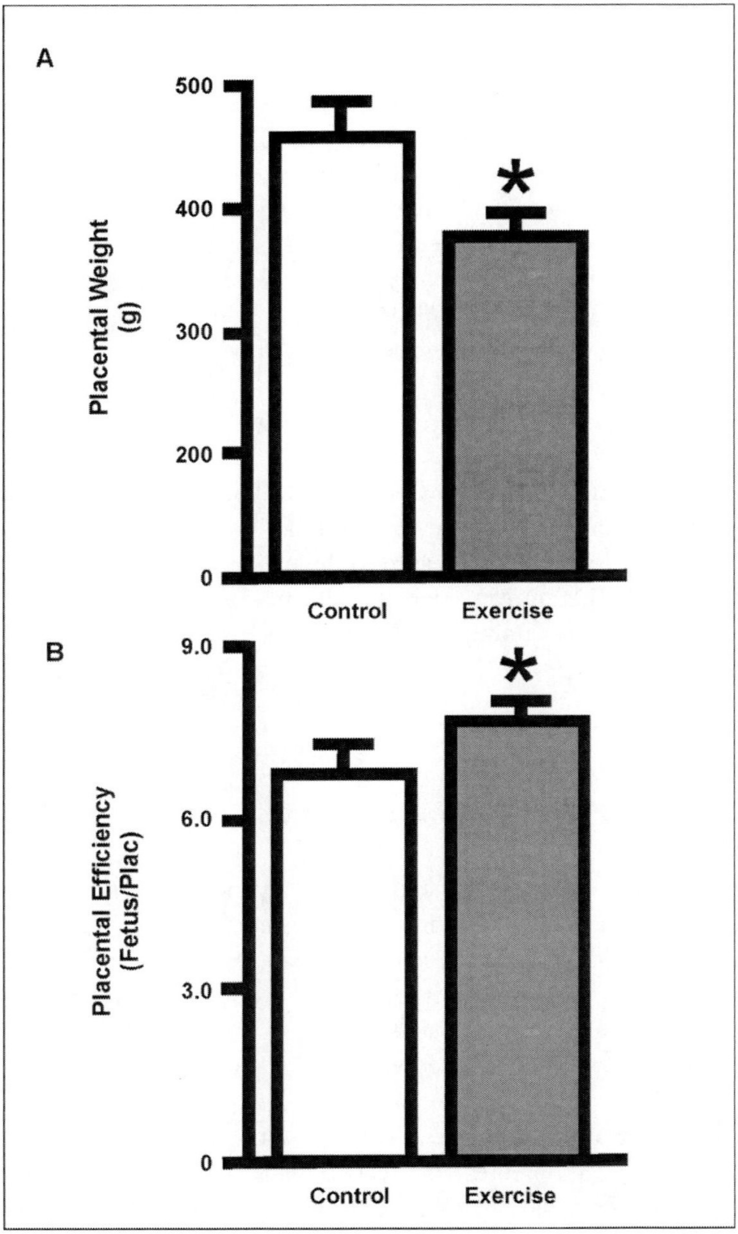

Figure 7. Effects of exercise on placental weight (panel A) and placental efficiency (panel B). Placental weight was decreased in the exercise trained compared to the non-exercised while placental efficiency was increased in the exercise group. Data are expressed as mean ± SEM. (*$p < 0.05$, as compared with control value).

Respiratory Complexes Activity

Activity of complex I-III of the mitochondrial respiratory chain was increased by 29% in submitochondrial membranes obtained from human placenta of exercised women, as compared with control subjects ($p<0.05$) (Figure 6A). Also, significant increases of 45% and 21%, ($p<0.05$) were observed in complexes II-III (Figure 6B) and in complex IV respectively in submitochondrial membranes from exercised women, as compared with the controls (Figure 6C).

Maternal and Conceptus Morphometrics

Fetal weight (3013.2 ± 493.8 vs. 3133.3 ± 406.5 g) was not altered in the exercise trained compared to the non-exercise group. In contrast, placental (Figure 7A; $p<0.05$) weight decreased in the exercise trained compared to the non-exercised. Furthermore, placental efficiency was increased (Figure 7B; $p<0.05$) in the exercise trained. There was no difference in the number of cotyledons (12.5 ± 0.5 vs. 12 ± 1.0) between the exercise and non-exercise groups.

Discussion

The present study reveals several interesting and novel findings regarding maternal and placental adaptations to chronic exercise training during pregnancy. Exercise training during pregnancy led to a 2-fold increase in eNOS expression and a 4-fold increase in NO production in placental cytosol. Exercised women also showed 6% decreases in mitochondrial O_{2-} levels and 26% decreases in H_2O_2 production rate in placental mitochondria. NO generated by NOS has been demonstrated to contribute to the regulation of vascular tone by counteracting the actions of vasoconstrictors [29]. NOS in the placental villous vasculature also corresponds to the type III calcium-calmodulin-dependent endothelial isoform, and no such NOS was found in the cytotrophoblast layer or in small fetal blood capillaries of term placenta [30]. According to the present findings, a combined resistance and aerobic exercise training program leads to an increased eNOS expression and NO production in human placental tissue. Potentially, the underlying mechanisms may relate to an exercise induced increase in shear stress on the endothelial monolayer, in turn enhancing the activity of enzymes such as eNOS and extracellular superoxide dismutase and shifting the reactive oxygen balance toward the beneficial NO [31]. However, other vasoactive substances such as prostacyclin, or endothelium-derived hyperpolarizing factor (EDHF) could also be involved [1, 2]. It has been reported that exercise produces a state of hyperemia and an increase of blood flow and shear stress with a consequent increase in the production and bioactivity of NO [15, 16]. However, parallel or subsequent events are less clear, and whether the improvement in endothelium function induced by exercise during pregnancy observed in the present study has a beneficial effect in the prevention of these disorders (i.e., reduced risk of preeclampsia, diabetes or hypertension), is yet to be determined.

Placental function is critical to pregnancy outcome and to a healthy start to life for the offspring and hence an understanding of events and the effects of strategies that could improve outcomes could have significant translational consequences. Exercise during pregnancy appears to be beneficial to the maternal-fetal unit and may prevent the occurrence of maternal disorders. The exact reason for this remains unclear but, it is likely that endurance training induced mitochondrial biogenesis, a typical response for adaptation to physical activity. It has been described that exercise modulates mitochondrial content in healthy, lean, normal individuals.

Human placenta can manifest considerable plasticity of mitochondrial content, adapting to match energy demands of physical activity [32]. Indeed, some of the age-associated alterations found in mitochondrial activity can be the result of a reduction in the level of voluntary physical activity as individuals age [33, 34].

Some of the exercise-induced changes serve as regulating signals for the adjustment of the rate of ATP synthesis to increased energy demand [35]. However, challenged intracellular homeostasis during acute exercise may not only affect the respiration rate of mitochondria, but may also elicit lasting alterations in the intrinsic properties of mitochondrial function [36].

The placenta generates reactive oxygen species which may contribute to the oxidative stress seen even in normal pregnancy, but this is increased in pregnancies complicated by pre-eclampsia, IUGR and gestational diabetes where elevated oxidative and nitrative stress have been clearly documented [37]. Nitrative stress is the covalent modification of proteins and DNA by H_2O_2 formed by the interaction of O_{2-} and NO [38]. In the present study, reactive oxygen species O_{2-} and H_2O_2 were significantly diminished in human placental mitochondria from exercised women as compared with control subjects, suggesting that chronic exercise training results in a lower level of oxidative stress. Studies by Bo et al., [39] showed that during prolonged exercise, UCP2 mRNA expression and activity in rat heart can be upregulated, thereby reducing cross-membrane $\Delta\psi$ and reactive oxygen species production. One of the important effects of increased UCP2 expression is to decrease the generation of oxygen free radicals in the mitochondria. These results were in agreement with studies by Venditti et al., [40] who found that succinate-supported H_2O_2 release was higher in skeletal muscle from trained rats in both State 4 and State 3, while training did not affect mitochondrial oxygen consumption with both complex-I- and complex II-linked substrates.

We also report that exercise training during pregnancy was associated with a decreased placental weight, but an increased placental efficiency (fetal weight: placental weight). Previous studies have reported a wide range of effects of chronic exercise before and during pregnancy on conceptus weight in both humans [13,14] and rats [41]. The underlying differences between these observations remain unclear but the wide variation in the amounts and types of exercise are likely contributing factors. Further studies are needed to determine if other indices of placenta function such as transport of amino acids and vascular density are improved by exercise training.

More laboratory based studies and clinical trials are needed to confirm and elaborate the effects of aerobic and resistance exercises as the small sample size, warrants caution in the interpretation of the results. Nevertheless, these results may offer a plausible explanation for previous reports showing a decreased incidence of preeclampsia in woman participating in exercise training [42] and are consistent with findings from previous studies in other tissues [43].

Our findings do further strengthen the notion that moderate, carefully supervised exercise can be safely performed by pregnant women until the end of pregnancy even if they were previously sedentary. As a general conclusion, endurance training can preserve mitochondrial function, increases eNOS expression and NO production and decrease reactive oxygen species generation at the mitochondrial respiratory chain in placental mitochondria. Increases in complexes I-IV activities in human placental mitochondria can help to improve mitochondrial respiratory activity in trained subjects.

As a general conclusion, regular exercise training during the second half of pregnancy and decreases reactive oxygen species generation in the mitochondrial respiratory chain in placental mitochondria. This finding provides a pathophysiologic framework for the elucidation of the positive effects of exercise on placental human and demonstrates the therapeutic potential of exercise training to improve fetal oxygenation and in turn potentially reduce risk of gestational disorders associated with impaired endothelial and/or mitochondrial function.

Funding

This study was funded by Instituto Colombiano para el Desarrollo de la Ciencia y la Tecnología "Francisco José de Caldas" COLCIENCIAS (Grant N° 1106-45921540). Robinson Ramírez-Vélez received a grant from Instituto Colombiano para el Desarrollo de la Ciencia y la Tecnología "Francisco José de Caldas") to do a doctorate (Grant Colciencias/Icetex N° 067/2002). The funders had no role in study design, data collection and analysis, decision to publish, or preparation of the manuscript.

Competing Interests

The authors declare that they have no competing interests.

References

[1] Sierra-Laguado J, Garcia RG, Lopez-Jaramillo P. Flow mediated dilatation of the brachial artery in pregnancy. *Int. J. Gynecol. Obstet.* 2006;93:60-61.

[2] Brown CM, Garovic VD. Mechanisms and management of hypertension in pregnant women. *Curr. Hypertens Rep*. 2011;13:338-46.

[3] Wisdom SJ, Wilson R, McKillop JH, Walker JJ. Antioxidant systems in normal pregnancy and in pregnancy-induced hypertension. *Am. J. Obstet. Gynecol.* 1991;165(6 Pt 1):1701-4.

[4] Myatt L, Cui X. Oxidative stress in the placenta. *Histochem. Cell Biol.* 2004;122:369-82.

[5] Oostdam N, van Poppel MN, Eekhoff EM, Wouters MG, van Mechelen W. Design of FitFor2 study: the effects of an exercise program on insulin sensitivity and plasma glucose levels in pregnant women at high risk for gestational diabetes. *BMC Pregnancy Childbirth*. 2009 5;9:1.

[6] Hegaard HK, Pedersen BK, Nielsen BB, Damm P. Leisure time physical activity during pregnancy and impact on gestational diabetes mellitus,

pre-eclampsia, preterm delivery and birth weight: a review. *Acta. Obstet. Gynecol. Scand.* 2007;86:1290-6.
[7] ACOG Committee Opinion No. 267. Exercise during pregnancy and the postpartum period American college of obstetricians and gynecologists. *Obstet. Gynecol.* 2002;99:171-3.
[8] Jackson MRP, Gott SJ, Ritchie JW, Clapp III JF. The effects of maternal aerobic exercise on human placental development: placental volumetric composition and surface areas. *Placenta.* 1995;16:179-91.
[9] Genest DS, Falcao S, Gutkowska J, Lavoie JL. Impact of exercise training on preeclampsia: potential preventive mechanisms. *Hypertension.* 2012;60:1104-9.
[10] Fortner RT, Pekow PS, Whitcomb BW, Sievert LL, Markenson G, Chasan-Taber L. Physical activity and hypertensive disorders of pregnancy among Hispanic women. Med. Sci. Sports *Exerc.* 2011;43:639-46.
[11] Han S, Middleton P, Crowther CA. Exercise for pregnant women for preventing gestational diabetes mellitus. *Cochrane Database Syst. Rev.* 2012;7:CD009021.
[12] Clapp III JF. Influence of endurance exercise and diet on human placental development and fetal growth. *Placenta.* 2006;27:527-34.
[13] Clapp III JF, Kim H, Burciu B, Lopez B. Beginning regular exercise in early pregnancy: effect on fetoplacental growth. *Am. J. Obstet. Gynecol.* 2000;183:1484-8.
[14] Bergmann A, Zygmunt M, Clapp III JF. Running throughout pregnancy: effect on placental villous vascular volume and cell proliferation. *Placenta.* 2004;25:694-8.
[15] Ramírez-Vélez R, Aguilar de Plata AC, Mosquera-Escudero M, Echeverri I, Ortega JG, Salazar B, et al., Influence of regular aerobic exercise on Endothelium-Dependent Vasodilation and Cardio-respiratory Fitness in pregnant women. *J. Obstet. Gynaecol. Res.* 2011;37:1601-8.
[16] Hood DA. Invited Review: contractile activity-induced mitochondrial biogenesis in skeletal muscle. *J. Appl. Physiol.* 2001;90:1137-57.
[17] Hood DA. Mechanisms of exercise-induced mitochondrial biogenesis in skeletal muscle. *Appl. Physiol. Nutr. Metab.* 2009;34:465-72.
[18] Kang C, O'Moore KM, Dickman JR, Ji LL. Exercise activation of muscle peroxisome proliferator-activated receptor-gamma coactivator-1alpha signaling is redox sensitive. *Free Radic. Biol. Med.* 2009; 47:1394-1400.

[19] Ramirez-Velez R, Aguilar AC, Mosquera M, Garcia RG, Reyes LM, Lopez-Jaramillo P. Clinical trial to assess the effect of physical exercise on endothelial function and insulin resistance in pregnant women. *Trials.* 2009;10:104.

[20] Institute of Medicine of the National Academies Committee on the Scientific Evaluation of Dietary Reference Intakes. Dietary Reference Intakes: The Essential Reference for Dietary Planning and Assessment. Washington (DC): The National Academies Press; 2006. pp. 87–94.

[21] Martinez F, Meaney A, Espinosa-Garcia MT, Pardo JP, Uribe A, Flores-Herrera O. Characterization of the F1F0-ATPase and the tightly-bound ATPase activities in submitochondrial particles from human term placenta. *Placenta.* 1996;17:345-50.

[22] Martinez F, Espinosa-Garcia T, Flores-Herrera O, Pardo JP. Respiratory control induced by ATP in human term placental mitochondria. *Placenta.* 1993;14:321-31.

[23] Boveris A, D'Amico G, Lores-Arnaiz S, Costa LE. Enalapril increases mitochondrial nitric oxide synthase activity in heart and liver. *Antioxid Redox. Signal.* 2003;5: 691-7.

[24] Boveris A. Determination of the production of superoxide radicals and hydrogen peroxide in mitochondria. *Methods Enzymol.* 1984;105: 429-35.

[25] Boveris A, Costa LE, Cadenas E, Poderoso JJ. Regulation of mitochondrial respiration by adenosine diphosphate, oxygen, and nitric oxide. *Methods Enzymol.* 1999;301:188-98.

[26] Yonetani T. Cytochrome oxidase: beef heart. *Methods Enzymol.* 1967;10:3332-35.

[27] Lowry OH, Rosebrough NJ, Farr AL, Randall RJ. Protein measurement with the Folin phenol reagent. *J. Biol. Chem.* 1951;193:265-75.

[28] Lores-Arnaiz S, D'Amico G, Czerniczyniec A, Bustamante J, Boveris A. Brain mitochondrial nitric oxide synthase: in vitro and in vivo inhibition by chlorpromazine. *Arch. Biochem. Biophys.* 2004;430:170-7.

[29] Winfried G. Rossmanith, Ulrike Hoffmeister, Sonja Wolfahrt, Bernhard Kleine, Marc McLean, et al., Expression and functional analysis of endothelial nitric oxide synthase (eNOS) in human placenta. *Mol. Hum. Reprod.* 1999; 5:487-94.

[30] Myatt L, Brockman DE, Eis AL, Pollock JS. Immunohistochemical localization of nitric oxide synthase in the human placenta. *Placenta.* 1993;14:487-95.

[31] Laufs U, Werner N, Link A, Endres M, Wassmann S, Jürgens K, et al., Physical training increases endothelial progenitor cells, inhibits neointima formation, and enhances angiogenesis. *Circulation.* 2004;109:220-6.
[32] Barrientos A, Casademont J, Rotig A, Miro O, Urbano-Marquez A, Rustin P, Cardellach F. Absence of relationship between the level of electron transport chain activities and aging in human skeletal muscle. *Biochem. Biophys. Res. Commun.* 1996;229:536-39.
[33] Hegaard HK, Pedersen BK, Nielsen BB, Damm P. Leisure time physical activity during pregnancy and impact on gestational diabetes mellitus, pre-eclampsia, preterm delivery and birth weight: a review. Acta Obstet. *Gynecol. Scand.* 2007;86:1290-6.
[34] Jackson MRP, Gott SJ, Ritchie JW, Clapp III JF. The effects of maternal aerobic exercise on human placental development: placental volumetric composition and surface areas. *Placenta.* 1995;16:179-91.
[35] Tonkonogi M, Walsh B, Svensson M, Sahlin K. Mitochondrial function and antioxidative defence in human muscle: effects of endurance training and oxidative stress. *J. Physiol.* 2000;528:2379-88.
[36] Kay L, Nicolay K, Wieringa B, Saks V, Wallimann T. Direct evidence for the control of mitochondrial respiration by mitochondrial creatine kinase in oxidative muscle cells in situ. *J. Biol. Chem.* 2000;275:6937-44.
[37] Wang Y, Walsh SW. Increased superoxide generation is associated with decreased superoxide dismutase activity and mRNA expression in placental trophoblast cells in pre-eclampsia. Placenta. 2001;22:206-12.
[38] Myatt L. Review: Reactive oxygen and nitrogen species and functional adaptation of the placenta. *Placenta.* 2010;31 Suppl:S66-9.
[39] Bo H, Jiang N, Ma G, Qu J, Zhang G, Cao D, et al., Regulation of mitochondrial uncoupling respiration during exercise in rat heart: role of reactive oxygen species (ROS) and uncoupling protein 2. *Free Radic. Biol. Med.* 2008;44:1373-81.
[40] Venditti P, Masullo P, Di Meo S. Effect of training on H(2)O(2) release by mitochondria from rat skeletal muscle. *Arch. Biochem. Biophys.* 1999;372:315-20.
[41] Gilbert JS, Banek CT, Bauer AJ, Gingery A, Dreyer HC. Placental and vascular adaptations to exercise training before and during pregnancy in the rat. *Am. J. Physiol. Regul. Integr. Comp. Physiol.* 2012 1;303: R520-6.

[42] Yeo S, Davidge S, Ronis DL, Antonakos CL, Hayashi R, O'Leary S. A comparison of walking versus stretching exercises to reduce the incidence of preeclampsia: a randomized clinical trial. *Hypertens Pregnancy.* 2008;27:113–130.

[43] Ramírez-Vélez R. Aerobic exercise training during pregnancy increases antioxidant status in nulliparous women: Secondary analysis of a controlled clinical trial. *Endocrinol. Nutr.* 2013;60:279-81.

In: Fetal Development
Editor: Josiah Wilburn
ISBN: 978-1-63117-069-0

Chapter 4

MATERNAL MELAMINE AND FETAL DEVELOPMENT

***Ching Yan Chu*[1,*], *Kwok Pui Fung*[2,†] *and Chi Chiu Wang*[1,2,‡]**

[1]Department of Obstetrics and Gynaecology, [2]School of Biomedical Sciences, The Chinese University of Hong Kong, Shatin, New Territories, Hong Kong

ABSTRACT

Melamine is widely used in paint, plastic, textile and paper industries for its shrink-resistant, water-repellent, stain-repellent, and fire-retardant properties. It has made itself ill-famous by appearing in animal feeds and dairy products, affecting thousands of pets, farm animals and human infants in the early 21st century. The conventional Kjehdahl test for crude protein measurement in foodstuffs was deceived by the high-nitrogen content of melamine, disclosing the compound as an economically motivated adulteration. However, the presence of melamine in food leached from food-contacting table 'melawares' and food containers with

* E-mail: nina_chu@cuhk.edu.hk.
† E-mail: kpfung@cuhk.edu.hk.
‡ Corresponding Author: Prof. WANG Chi Chiu, Department of Obstetrics and Gynaecology, The Chinese University of Hong Kong, c/o 1st Floor, Block E, Prince of Wales Hospital, Shatin, New Territories, Hong Kong. Tel: (852) 2632 2810. Fax: (852) 2636 0008. Email: ccwang@cuhk.edu.hk.

melamine-formaldehyde coating has also been recognised as an unintentional contamination in our daily food chain. Nephrotoxicity due to the high-dose melamine intoxication from deliberate contamination have been well characterised. Histopathological findings of melamine crystal damaging the urinary system included renal tubular dilation, inflammation and carcinoma. Recent data on melamine reproductive and developmental toxicity are also identified. The maternal physiological changes during pregnancy may alter the toxicokinetic profile of melamine, which may in turn pose more serious threats to the affected mothers and their foetuses than to the non-pregnant adults. On the other hand, the developing embryo and foetal organs, not limited to kidneys, may also be vulnerable points of melamine toxicity. Prenatal exposure of melamine from the maternal intake of the contaminated pregnancy formulae and postnatal intake of adulterated infant formulae can perturb the development of the kidney, which the effect may carry on to the later stages of life. In this chapter, the reproductive and development toxicity of melamine will be addressed in details.

1. INTRODUCTION

1.1. Chemistry of Melamine

Melamine (IUPAC ID: 1,3,5-Triazine-2,4,6-triamine) is an aromatic amine that lacks functional groups. It appears as white crystalline powder with a low solubility in water, i.e.3.2 g/L at room temperature. It is manufactured from dehydrating urea at a temperature higher than 250°C; cyanuric acid is an intermediate of the reaction (Kinoshita, 1953) (Kinoshita, 1954). The majority of the melamine manufactured is reacted to form thermosetting resin for laminates, protective coatings, moulding compounds, textile finishes and paper coatings with applications in a large variety of industries, e.g. textile, tableware, furniture and automotive. Lesser is used to manufacture melamine crystal or salts for flame retardant or moisture-resistant applications, cleansing and etching agents, etc (European Chemical News, 2004).

1.2. Metabolism of Melamine

In our daily life, the main route of melamine exposure is oral intake; however, it is never a food or a drug to human as it has neither nutritional nor pharmacological values. It is not metabolised in mammalian cells (Mast et al,

1983; Panesar et al, 2010) but certain species of bacteria are capable of doing so.

Bacteria, including *Pseudomonas* sp (Jutzi et al, 1982; Eaton & Karns, 1991; Cheng et al, 2005), *Klebsiella terragena* (Hapeman et al, 1995; Shelton et al, 1997) and *Nocardioides* sp (Takagi et al, 2012), *Pseudomonas putida* KT2440 (Cheng et al, 2005), *Escherichia coli* K-12 MG1655 (Cheng et al, 2005), *Micrococcus* sp MF-1 (El-Sayed et al, 2006) and *Rhodococcus* sp strain Mel (Dodge et al, 2012) are able to degrade melamine into its interacting metabolites, namely, ammeline, ammelide and cyanuric acid (Table 1).

Triazine compounds like atrazine and cyromazine are employed as herbicides and insecticides (Yokley et al, 2000; Wackett et al, 2002). A family of Atz/Trz genes has been identified in microbes, which are responsible in the degradation and metabolism of the *s*-triazine compounds. Complete biodegradation of *s*-triazine ends up as ammonia and carbon dioxide, with melamine as an intermediate (Lim et al, 1990; Yokley et al, 2000; Wackett et al, 2002).

Melamine aminohydrolase and *s*-triazine hydrolase (TrzA) were identified in *Pseudomonas* sp strain NRRLB-12227 and soil *Rhodococcus* sp strain Mel, respectively, which can convert melamine into ammeline (Eaton & Karns, 1991; Dodge et al, 2012); ammeline aminohydrolase in *Pseudomonas* sp strain NRRLB-12227, guanine deaminase in *Pseudomonas putida* KT2440, *Escherichia coli* K-12 MG1655, *Bradyrhizobium japonicum* USDA 110, and melamine deaminase (TriA) in *Rhodococcus* sp strain Mel convert ammeline into ammelide (Eaton & Karns, 1991; Seffernick et al, 2010; Dodge et al, 2012); ammelide aminohydrolase in *Pseudomonas* sp strain NRRLB-12227, *n*-isopropylammelide aminohydrolase (AtzC) in *Pseudomonas* sp strain ADP and *Nocardioides* sp strain ATD6 convert ammelide into cyanuric acid (Eaton & Karns, 1991; Seffernick et al, 2002; Takagi et al, 2012); cyanuric acid aminohydrolase (TrzD) in *Pseudomonas* sp strain NRRLB-12227 converts cyanuric acid into biuret (Eaton & Karns, 1991). Biuret aminohydrolase and urease convert biuret into ammonia and CO_2 with urea as an intermediate (Eaton & Karns, 1991) while convertion by biuret hydrolase (AtzE) and allophanate hydrolase (AtzF) with allophanate as an intermediate (Cheng et al, 2005). *Pseudomonas* sp strain A, *Klebsiella terragena* strain DRS-1 and *Micrococcus* sp MF-1 also showed the ability to degrade melamine into ammonia and CO_2 (Jutzi et al, 1982; Hapeman et al, 1995; El-Sayed et al, 2006; Shelton et al, 1997).

Cyromazine → Melamine → Ammeline → Ammelide → Cyanuric Acid → Biuret → Urea → Ammonia + Carbon Dioxide.

Table 1. Bacterial degradation of melamine to ammonia and carbon dioxide

Microbes	Reaction	Enzyme	
Pseudomonas sp strain NRRLB-12227	Melamine → Ammeline	Melamine aminohydrolase	Eaton & Karns, 1991
Rhodococcus sp strain Mel	Melamine → Ammeline	*s*-Triazine hydrolase (TrzA)	Dodge et al, 2012.
Pseudomonas sp strain NRRLB-12227	Ammeline → Ammelide	Ammeline aminohydrolase (guanine deaminase)	Eaton & Karns, 1991
Pseudomonas putida KT2440, *Escherichia coli* K-12 MG1655, *Bradyrhizobium japonicum* USDA 110	Ammeline → Ammelide	Guanine deaminase	Seffernick et al, 2010.
Rhodococcus sp strain Mel	Ammeline → Ammelide	Melamine deaminase (TriA)	Dodge et al, 2012.
Pseudomonas sp strain NRRLB-12227	Ammelide → Cyanuric acid	Ammelide aminohydrolase (TrzC)	Eaton & Karns, 1991
Pseudomonas sp strain ADP	Ammelide → Cyanuric acid	Isopropylammelide aminohydrolase(AtzC)	Seffernick et al, 2002.
Nocardioides sp strain ATD6	Ammelide → Cyanuric acid	Isopropylammelide aminohydrolase(AtzC)	Takagi et al, 2012.
Pseudomonas sp strain NRRLB-12227	Cyanuric acid → Biuret	Cyanuric acid aminohydrolase (TrzD)	Eaton & Karns, 1991
Pseudomonas sp strain NRRLB-12227	Biuret → Urea	Biuret aminohydrolase	Eaton & Karns, 1991
Pseudomonas sp strain ADP, *Ralstonia pickettii* strain D, *Agrobacterium radiobacter* strain J14a	Biuret → Allophanate	Biuret hydrolase (AtzE)	Cheng et al, 2005.
Pseudomonas sp strain NRRLB-12227	Urea → $NH_3 + CO_2$	Urease	Eaton & Karns, 1991
Pseudomonas sp strain ADP, *Ralstonia pickettii* strain D, *Agrobacterium radiobacter* strain J14a	Allophanate → $NH_3 + CO_2$	Allophanate hydrolase (AtzF)	Cheng et al, 2005.
Pseudomonas sp strain A	Melamine →→ $NH_3 + CO_2$		Jutzi et al, 1982.
Klebsiella terragena strain DRS-1	Melamine →→ $NH_3 + CO_2$		Hapeman et al, 1995
Klebsiella terragena strain DRS-1	Melamine →→ $NH_3 + CO_2$		Shelton et al, 1997.
Micrococcus sp MF-1	Melamine formaldehyde →→ $NH_3 + CO_2$		El-Sayed et al, 2006.

Although mammalian cells lack the enzymes for metabolism and degradation of melamine (Mast et al, 1983; Panesar et al, 2010), scientific evidences have shown that melamine can still be converted to its metabolites inside the mammalian bodies. It is done so by the microbiota residing in the rumens of the ruminants and in the gut of the monogastric species. By the administration of antibiotics which suppresses the microbial activity, conversion of melamine to its metabolites was suppressed in a rat study. The microbes identified in the experiment included *Klebsiella terrigena*, *Klebsiella pneumonia* and *Klebsiella planticola* (Zheng et al, 2013). *Klebsiella* sp are also present in the guts of human and pig (Conlan et al, 2012; Dai et al, 2012); therefore, conversion of melamine into its metabolites is possible to occur in different mammals.

1.3. Melamine Deceiving the Kjeldahl Test

With the help of the microbiota, melamine, its industrial precursor – urea, and its metabolite – biuret are often used as the nitrogen filler in the animal feed for the ruminents (Barboza & Barrionuevo, 2007). The molecular formula of melamine, C3H6N6, shows that 67% of its weight is from nitrogen. Despite its relatively environmentally stable property, the structure dissociates in destructive reductions like the Kjeldahl method and forms ammonium ions. The conversion of melamine to this simple molecule has been playing a critical trick in the deception of the humble food test.

The Kjeldahl test is a simple and conventional method for crude protein determination in the food industry. Regardless of the source of the nitrogen atom in a compound or food source, all nitrogen will result in ammonium ion, which will then be back titrated for quantitation (Dakin & Dudley, 1914). As a result, non-proteineous source of nitrogen can deceive the conventional quantitation of protein.

Degradation:	$Sample + H_2SO_4 \rightarrow (NH_4)_2SO_4 + CO_2 + SO_2 + H_2O$
Liberation of ammonia:	$(NH_4)_2SO_4 + 2NaOH \rightarrow Na_2SO_4 + 2H_2O + 2NH_3$
Capture of ammonia:	$B(OH)_3 + H_2O + NH_3 \rightarrow NH_4^+ + B(OH)_4^-$
Back-titration:	$B(OH)_3 + H_2O + Na_2CO_3 \rightarrow NaHCO_3 + NaB(OH)_4 + CO_2 + H_2O$

Since a single molecule of melamine contains 6 nitrogen atoms, while a single amine group in a protein contains only 1 nitrogen atom, weight by weight, melamine costs much less to produce the same positive result in the non-discriminative Kjeldahl test. This property of melamine was dishonestly exploited so as to falsely boost the protein content in foodstuff.

2. ADULTERATION

2.1. Melamine Incident

In 2007, sickening and death of thousands of family pets were reported around the North America (Table 2). These animals had the clinical presentations of inappetence, vomiting, polyuria, polydipsia, lethargy and azotemia in the affected animals (Cianciolo et al, 2008). Pathological findings confirmed that these animals suffered from acute kidney injury (AKI, previously known as acute renal failure). More than 8000 deaths of cats and dogs were reported by the US Food and Drug Administration (US FDA) (Goldman & Lee, 2007). Food poisoning may be the reason for such a wide spread of disease. Melamine was not the first suspect, but the rodenticide aminopterin. Later, presence of melamine was confirmed in the imported Chinese wheat gluten that was used as the main plant protein source for the affected pet food manufactured by the Menu Foods, the biggest manufacturer at that time (Goodman, 2007).

Contamination of animal feeds for pets and farm animals can go back in time to 2004. Necropsy from the affected pets in 2004 and 2007 showed common features for suspecting the same culprit: distal tubular necrosis and intra-tubular crystals in all of the renal specimens. Some of them showed signs of chronic tubulointerstitial nephritis while other observations included mild anisokaryosis, focal proliferation of tubular epithelial cells, renal interstitial fibrosis, lymphoplasmacytic inflammation. Away from the urinary system, oral ulcers, gastric and pulmonary mineralisation were also reported (Jeong et al, 2006; Brown et al, 2007).

In about the same period of time, some Spanish and Thai farms suffered from sickening and deaths of post-weaning piglets. Intratubular, round, yellow-brown crystals with radiating striations, dilation of the proximal and the distal tubules (Nilubol et al, 2009), severe interstitial nephritis and fibrosis with crystal deposition were found in the affected piglets but the damage to the renal tubular epithelial cells was milder in piglets than in cats and dogs (González et al, 2009). A Thai laboratory report revealed that the pig feed was contaminated with an average of 3209 mg/kg of melamine with the presence of ammeline and cyanuric acid. Melamine accumulated in the pig kidney in a concentration as high as 7692 mg/kg (Nilubol et al, 2009).

Deaths of the animal victims have not stopped the spread of melamine from contaminating food articles. In 2008, sudden increase in paediatric AKI, nephrolithiasis and urolithiasis were reported in China. The majority of the victims required hospitalisation and many of them were under the age of 3 (Hu et al, 2010; Lu et al, 2011; Shi et al, 2012).

Table 2. Half-lives and suggested withdrawal time of melamine in various food animals

Time	Country	Species	Contaminants	Symptoms	
2003 – 2006	Spain	Pig	Melamine, cyanuric acid, ammeline, ammelide	Enlarged kidneys, nephroliths, chronic inflammation	González et al, 2009
2004	Korea	Dog	Melamine, cyanuric acid	Nephroliths, uremia, necrosis and calcification of renal tubules	Jeong et al, 2006; Brown et al, 2007
2004	Taiwan	Dog	Not identified	Kidney failure	Brown et al, 2007
2007	Thailand	Pig	Melamine, cyanuric acid, ammeline	Yellowish, swollen kidney, nephroliths, tubular epithelial degeneration, necrosis of renal tubules	Nilubol et al, 2009
2007	North America	Dog, cat	Melamine, cyanuric acid	Uremia, renal tubular lesions, nephroliths, interstitial fibrosis, inflammation	Brown et al, 2007; Cianciolo et, 2008
2008	Italy	Dog	Melamine	Uremia, severe nephrotoxicosis, uroliths, interstitial fibrosis, inflammation	Cocchi et al, 2010
2008	China	Human infants	Melamine	Acute renal injurty, hydronephrosis, uroliths, nephroliths, haematuria	Xinhua Net, 2007; Shang et al, 2012; Shi et al, 2012; Sun et al, 2009; Chen et al, 2010; Zhang et al, 2009; Wang et al, 2009
2008	Hong Kong, Macau, Taiwan, etc	Human	Melamine		Lam et al, 2008; Wu et al, 2010; Kong et al, 2011
2010	China		Melamine		BBC News, 2010

The numbers of the affected children was estimated to be 30,000,000, sickened 300,000 and death 6 (Xinhua Net, 2007). Melamine was later found to have entered the food chain in the milk delivered from farmland; other foodstuffs with milk as ingredient were also contaminated.

Under the efficiency of global trading, food laced with the notorious contaminant spread quickly throughout the world. The mostly affected areas included Hong Kong, Macau, Taiwan, Singapore, Japan, South Korea and Australia; the problematic foodstuff spanned from infant formulae, eggs, chocolates and some other snack. Although the milk formulae and food were less tainted in these countries, the affected infants and young children also suffered from renal and urinary stone and crystals, haematuria and hydronephrosis (Lam et al, 2008; Wang et al, 2009; Shi et al, 2012). In order to stop the epidemic, many food articles were pulled from the shelves worldwide together with the problematic milk formulae. Many countries even issued import ban of dairy products and snacks from China. The US FDA also opened her first office outside the US in her history, i.e. in Beijing, China.

2.2. Intentional Adulteration

For the high content of nitrogen in melamine and the incapability of the Kjeldahl test in discriminating the proteineous and the non-proteineous nitrogen sources, melamine was used to boost up the 'nitrogen content' in food. The comparatively higher nitrogen content of melamine makes it even more attractive than urea and biuret to be nitrogen filler in animal feeds, which the nitrogen content account for 47% and 41% of the molecular mass.

Lacing melamine in animal feeds and milk for human consumption is obviously economically motivated: less wheat, rice or cow's milk are needed to produce the same amount of protein to meet the international standard for food trade, which is set by the Codex Alimentarius Commission, e.g., the protein content in an infant formula prepared ready for consumption shall contain 1.8 – 3.0 g/100 kcal (Codex Alimentarius Commission, 2011).

In the 2008 Chinese outbreak in human consumed food articles, 69 batches of milk products produced by 22 companies were detected with the existence of melamine (WHO, 2009). The amount of melamine detected in the infant formulae at that period of time was 0.09 – 619 mg/kg (EFSA, 2008), while the worst adulterated ones were the Sanlu infant formulae, i.e. 4700 mg/kg of melamine co-contaminated with 6.3 mg/kg of cyanuric acid (Wu et al, 2009b; Shi et al, 2012). Recall of infant formulae was issued. The Sanlu company itself sealed off 2176 tonnes of the adulterated milk powder and recalled another 8210 tonnes that had been delivered to the market (Xinhua Net, 2008).The melamine levels detected in food sold in Hong Kong ranged from 1.4 – 68 mg/kg. The highest was measured in a Chinese-made chocolate filled biscuit, while the legal limit in Hong Kong was 2.5 mg/kg at that time (CFS HK, 2009). The melamine content of some of the products exceeded the legal limit.

Unfortunately, some of the confiscated melamine laced milk products re-entered the market 2 years later. More than 170 tonnes of those products was once again recalled (BBC News, 2010). Some were sold to farms to prepare feed to piglets, in a concentration 515 times higher than the Chinese safety standards (Jian & Raina, 2011). Animal feeds for fish and poultry were also found with the addition of melamine (Barboza & Barrionuevo, 2007; Barboza, 2008).

From the toxicology study of melamine, one may notice that the contamination by melamine alone may not cause problems as serious as seen with the co-contamination by cyanuric acid and other metabolites like ammeline and ammelide. The solubility of melamine in water is 3.2 g/L but once it forms complex with cyanuric acid, the solubility almost drops to zero. In the 2007 Spanish piglet incident, very high levels of ammelide, ammeline, melamine and cyanuric acid were detected in the heavily adulterated pig feed, ranging from 0.39 – 0.92% (ammelide), 0.2 – 0.34% (ammeline), 0.092 – 0.29% (melamine) and 0.022 – 0.091% (cyanuric acid) in those pig feed (González et al, 2009). These intentional contamination incidents of human or animal food have caused great economic loss and medical expenses.

2.3. Unintentional Adulteration

Unintentional adulteration is more difficult to quantify and to access the risks. Sources of the unintentional adulteration can be divided into bioaccumulation in food sources, migration from the food contact materials and environmental contamination.

2.3.1. Bioaccumulation in Food Sources

Feeding food animals with melamine-tainted fodder not only causes morbidity and mortality of the animals, but the contaminant accumulated in the animals will also travel up in the food chain and reach the top-level user, i.e. human, as the secondary poisoning. As reported from most of toxicokinetic studies, half-life of melamine is short but variations can be found between different organs and different species of animals. Like the application of pesticides, a withdrawal time should be given for the sufficient removal of the contaminant from the food before serving them on dining tables.

Generally speaking, half-life of orally administered melamine in plasma was around 2.5 hours in studies in rats and co-administration with cyanuric acid tripled the half-life of melamine (Pang et al, 2013; Jacob et al, 2012). However, half-life of melamine can be very different among different species and tissues (Table 3). Half-life of melamine in pig was 4 hours, probably due to the slower renal clearance (Baynes et al, 2008); half-life of melamine in goat was 11 hours due to the slow absorbance in the rumens (Baynes et al, 2010). Withdrawal time of melamine in pig predicted by a physiologically based pharmacokinetic study was around 21 hours (Buur et al, 2008).

On the contrary, a much longer 7-day withdrawal period was recommended in broiler chicken (Lü et al, 2009). Half-life of melamine in plasma and muscle of catfish and rainbow trout were 1.5 and 3.5 days respectively (Reimschuessel et al, 2010; Stine et al, 2012). The authors suggested a longer withdrawal time should be beneficial for the safe use of fish as human food, which may be as long as 1 month (Reimschuessel et al, 2010).

Besides meat, farm animals also produce egg and milk for human consumption. Melamine was detected in eggs of duck fed with melamine-laced fodder and remained at a high level in the 21-day feeding period. With the half-life of 0.7 day, the accumulated contaminant can be removed by promptly withdrawing the adulterated feed (Gao et al, 2010).

Table 3. Events of global melamine incidents

Species	Organ	Half-Life	Withdrawal Time	Reference
Pig	Plasma	4.07 h	28 h	Baynes et al, 2008
Pig	Muscle	N/A	21 h	Buur et al, 2008
Cow	Milk	N/A	152 h	Cruywagen et al, 2009
Goat	Plasma	11.12 h	60 h	Baynes et al, 2010
Catfish	Serum	1.62 days	7 days	Stine et al, 2012
Rainbow Trout	Serum	3.67 days	14 days	Stine et al, 2012
Catfish	Serum	1.5 days	7 days	Reimschuessel et al, 2010
Rainbow Trout	Serum	3.62 days	14 days	Reimschuessel et al, 2010
Chicken	Muscle	N/A	7 days	Lü et al, 2009

Melamine appeared in cow's milk 8 hours after the first ingestion and reached a maximum within 56 hours in a continuous daily intake of 17.1 g melamine/day per cow (Cruywagen et al, 2009). Unfortunately, a 5-day withdrawal time was not enough to bring the melamine down to level that is acceptable in the Codex Committee on Contaminants in Foods (CCCF) Guideline, i.e. 2.5 mg/kg for food other than liquid infant milk and powdered infant formulae (WHO, 2012). Maximum concentration of melamine appeared in goat's milk in 9.5 hours after the first administration but a lower level, single dose of melamine was able to be removed to an acceptable level in 60 hours (Baynes et al, 2010). For monogastric animals like rat, melamine concentration peak appeared earlier in 3 hours after a single bolus administration (Chu et al, 2010; Chan et al, 2011), but repeated dosing can lead to accumulation. The data on the lactational transfer of melamine in ruminants suggested the possibility of obtaining melamine from infant formulae produced by cow or goat, while that in small monogastric animal may help in understanding the same transfer observed in human breast feeding.

2.3.2. Migration from Food Contact Materials

Melamine is widely used in many food contact materials. The most common one is in the form of melamine-formaldehyde resin, which is known to be 'melamine-ware' or 'melaware'.

It is so welcomed by the public because of the resemblance of the appearance to ceramics but being much more durable and microwavable. Melamine can be used as coating of cans and glass bottle seals. It is also popular being a mild abrasive sponge that allows the reduction of detergent use in dish washing and kitchen cleaning.

Safety of melaware has been investigated in various parts of the world, sampling the authentic tableware sold in the market. Most of the commercially available melaware can be considered safe even treated with 3 – 4% acetic acid and heated up to 60 – 95°C (Sugita et al, 1990; Lund & Petersen, 2006; Bradley et al, 2010; Chik et al, 2011; CFS HK, 2010). Unfortunately, one study carried out in the UK in 2004 reported 10% of its tested samples had the melamine leaching above the legal specific migration limit, i.e. 30 mg/kg or 5.0 mg/dm^2 (Bradley et al, 2005). Health concern about the toxicity of the migrated formaldehyde is also a big issue of choosing melaware (Duong et al, 2011).

Manufacturers may have to re-think of some new and safe material for children's tableware.

2.3.3. Environmental Contamination

The insecticide cyromazine is viewed as the precursor of the majority of the melamine residue in soil (Root et al, 1996). Cyromazine can simply be photodegraded into melamine. The degradation product was detected in the cultivation of vegetables after cyromazine application as early as 2 hours (Lim et al, 1990) and the accumulation continued for at least 99 days (Patakioutas et al, 2007). The authors suggested melamine was accounted for 14 – 36% of the sum of the residual cyromazine and melamine in cultivation (Lim et al, 1990). Although generally *s*-triazines are believed to be degraded in soil via N-dealkylation, deamination and hydrolysis of the substituent on the C2 atom of the *s*-triazine ring (Erickson & Lee, 1989), degradation of the atypically substituted cyromazine into melamine can be carried out slowly by the bacterial community (Kontchou & Gschwind, 1999) or by plant tissues (Patakioutas et al, 2007).

3. Melamine and Pregnancy

3.1. Maternal Exposure to Melamine

In the last decade, the source of melamine contacted by human was mainly the contaminated milk. Infant formulae being the sole food source of the newborns nowadays, there is no doubt that the infants are the first to be affected. At the same time, popularity of pregnancy and lactating formulae are growing as a kind of nutrient supplement for the mothers. Contamination of these maternal formulae may also post risks of prenatal exposure to melamine and postnatal exposure through breast feeding.

Despite the fact that most of the toxicity investigations were carried out in adults, our recent works have shown evidences on the placental and the lactational transfer of melamine through the placenta and the mammary gland (Chu et al, 2010; Chan et al, 2011). After a single oral administration of melamine, the concentration of the contaminant in amniotic fluid peaked in around 3 hours (Chu et al, 2010; Chan et al, 2011) and it followed a dose-dependent fashion (Jingbin et al, 2010). A human term placenta allows melamine to pass through easily; as a result, melamine was detected in the foetal circulation in 5 min (Edelstam et al, 2007). Transfer of the maternally ingested melamine to the unborn foetus allows the foetal contact of the contaminant and may disturb the normal foetal development. Similar to the placental transfer, maximum concentration of melamine was detected in milk

3 hours after a single oral administration (Chu et al, 2010; Chan et al, 2011). Solely avoiding infant consuming the problematic infant formulae may not keep the vulnerable away from the risk. Breastfeeding can still be one of the routes of introducing the notorious contaminant if the mother takes in melamine through her daily diet.

3.2. Normal Physiological Changes During Pregnancy

Pregnancy requires a great physiological change in various systems in order to adapt to the need of the growing foetus. Changes may alter the maternal, placental and foetal contact to drugs or toxic substances in every aspect of absorption, distribution, metabolism and elimination (ADME).

3.2.1. Absorption

Absorption of substances under the changing physiology in pregnancy can be complicated. Many factors have to consider so as to predict the pharmaco- / toxico-kinetics and dynamics of a xenobiotic wisely. These factors include the gastrointestinal emptying, cardiac output, tidal volume of lung, etc.

When the chemical is administered through ingestion, its absorption will greatly depend on the motility of the gastrointestinal tract. Gastric pH and emptying time increase during pregnancy by 30 – 50% (Heikkilä & Erkkola, 1994). Thus, absorption of weak acids or molecules with small dissociation constant will become less efficient. On the contrary, the rate of absorption of weak bases and the time for the slowly absorbed xenobiotics will increase. The *p*Ka value of melamine is 5.0, suggesting it is a weak acid (Jang et al, 2009), which implies that the absorption of melamine should decrease in pregnant women. Experimental evidence was obtained in an animal model of rat. The time of detecting the maximum concentration of melamine increased insignificantly by 33% from the pre-pregnancy to late pregnancy, and the longest time needed was observed in mid-pregnancy (Chu et al, 2013).

Cardiac output increases by 30 – 50% towards the late pregnancy to meet the need of the placental circulation and the foetal growth but not to exceed the maternal tolerance. Accompanying the change in cardiac output, blood volume, heart rate, systemic blood pressure, vascular resistance and distribution of blood flow also have to acclimatise to the new need. Plasma volume increases by 45 – 60% by the 32nd week while the vascular resistance decreases by around 20% (Gei & Hankins, 2001). This resultant increase of peripheral blood flow may increase the absorption of xenobiotics.

If the xenobiotic is contacted through inhalation, the increased tidal volume during pregnancy can contribute to the change of the kinetics of the chemical. Increased tidal volume increases pulmonary distribution of gases and the alveolar mixing; thus the time to reach the alveolar steady state decreases (Mattison et al, 1991).

3.2.2. Distribution

Due to the tremendous increase in the blood volume and the amniotic fluid volume, the drug applied will be diluted to an extent that the usual dosage may not be able to produce the same therapeutic effect. This dilution effect is more prominent in the hydrophilic substances.

On the contrary, the accumulation of fat during pregnancy may delay the clearance of the lipophilic drugs. Reduction of plasma albumin concentration by 25% can have influence on the equilibrium of the bound and unbound portions of drugs (Krauer et al, 1984), where the unbound portion is usually the active portion. The availability and the clearance of the bound drugs can be lowered during pregnancy.

The uterine blood flow increases more than 10 times from early pregnancy to term, i.e. from 50 to 500 – 600 ml/min (Blackburn, 2003). The apparent volume of distribution of melamine changed during pregnancy: increased from pre-pregnancy to mid-pregnancy and decreased in the late pregnancy while the area-under-the-curve (AUC) of the melamine maternal serum profile increased from early to late pregnancy suggested melamine may be easier to be distributed to the periphery, and perhaps to the foetus, in the mid-gestation (Chu et al, 2010).

3.2.3. Metabolism

Hepatic First Pass

Right after absorption into blood, orally administered substances have to pass through the liver where many enzymes are present. The metabolism and elimination of these substances in the liver is called the first pass hepatic clearance.

Decrease in proportion of blood flow to the liver can lead to a decrease in clearance of xenobiotics or increase the retention of the toxic substances in the body. Substances with a low hepatic clearance rate are usually more affected by the physiological change during pregnancy. The reduced blood flow to the liver makes them less efficiently removed by the liver enzymes (Blackburn,

2003). In addition, the changes in the expression and the activity of these enzymes will also affect the resulting availability of the drugs or chemicals.

Kidney Metabolism

Kidney does not only passively remove substances by ultrafiltration, but it also possesses a number of enzymes that can convert xenobiotics into some other metabolites. Substances which can conjugate with glutathione (GSH) in kidney may produce renal toxicity by the resultant reactive thiolate anion, with the GSH *S*-conjugate, cysteine *S*-conjugate and *N*-acetylcysteine *S*-conjugate as the intermediates (Lash, 1994).

Similar to the hepatic metabolism, xenobiotics can either be detoxified or bioactivated in kidney. Toxicity of a xenobiotic will be complicated if the resultant metabolite is active and more toxic than the parent compound. Without known mammalian enzyme metabolising melamine, understanding of the melamine toxicity is simpler. About 90% of the [^{14}C]melamine administered to rat was excreted in urine within 24 hours, which the renal clearance rate was 2.5 ml/min (Mast et al, 1983).

More recent data suggest a portion of the rest of the melamine may be metabolised by the gut microbes and the consequent combination with the existing melamine accumulated in the kidney and bladder, making the higher radioactivity detected in those 2 organs than that in the plasma.

3.2.4. Elimination

Although drugs and chemicals can be removed by liver, lung and kidney, the latter is responsible for the majority of the elimination work. Most of the xenobiotics or their metabolites are excreted with urine *per se*, the change in the renal blood flowand the glomerular filtration rate (GFR) will determine the rate of clearance.

As an adaptation to the increase of the volume of body fluid, renal blow flow and GFR increase by 35 – 60% and 40 – 50%, respectively; urine output increases as a consequence. Decrease in GFR is noticed towards term, which may be up to 20%. Due to the increasing renal blood flow, human kidney has adopted some significant structural changes, e.g. dilatation of the renal calyces, pelvis and ureters, and increase in kidney length. As a result, pregnant women are more susceptible to infection and hydronephrosis (Blackburn, 2003). Experimentally, the apparent clearance of melamine dropped from early pregnancy towards term, the latter was about the same level of the pre-pregnant state, which suggested it was getting more difficult to remove melamine as pregnancy proceeded (Chu et al, 2013).

3.3. Melamine Toxicokinetic Characteristics During Pregnancy

The ADME of melamine changes obviously with the adaption of the maternal condition to the pregnancy. These changes are reflected from the toxicokinetic characteristics, more importantly the maximum concentration, the time of reaching the maximum concentration, the availability and the half-life of the contaminant. The toxicokinetic profiles of the non-pregnant and in late pregnancy of rat were similar. The lower availability of melamine during the early- and the mid-pregnancy is probably due to a less efficient absorption of the contaminant. The difference of the melamine toxicokinetic profiles during pregnancy reflects a complicated prediction of its toxicity to the developing foetus (Chu et al, 2013).

3.4. Maternal Renal Damage

Renal tubular necrosis / degeneration, dilation, hyaline disposition, crystals and recruitment of inflammatory cells were found in pregnant rat ingested melamine (Kim et al, 2011; Chu et al, unpublished data). Although these microscopic observations are similar to the non-pregnant subjects, pregnant rats may be more susceptible to the melamine nephrotoxicity with a higher incidence of crystal formation and tubular hyperplasia, which indicated the renal tubules were trying to regenerate after the toxic insult (Chu et al, unpublished data). This may be explained by the vigorous structural changes of the maternal kidney contribute to the higher rate of hydronephrosis in pregnant women (Rasmussen & Nielsen, 1988), as well as the higher GFR resulting in higher concentration of solutes in the renal tubules (Blackburn, 2003). These 2 factors working in concert may increase the severity of nephrotoxicity of melamine found in the pregnant rats.

The poorly water-soluble melamine can be easily concentrated in urine and crystallised in renal tubules. A study on the relationship between melamine-caused urinary bladder carcinogenesis and the formation of tumour suggested the irritation caused by the existence of the uroliths is the culprit, rather than the toxicity of the chemical itself (Ogasawara et al, 1995). Nephrolithiasis is rare in normal pregnancy but it can complicate the current and the future pregnancy including recurrent abortions, mild pre-eclampsia, gestational diabetes mellitus, caesarian delivery, pyelonephritis, urinary tract infection, hydronephrosis and hydroureter (Rosenberg et al, 2011). Current animal experiments on the developmental toxicity of melamine may not include some of these obstetric complication observations, but this study may give insights to the management of melamine-affected pregnancies.

4. MELAMINE AND FOETAL DEVELOPMENT

4.1. Placenta and Pathology

Placenta is a place for the foetal anchorage, gaseous exchange, nutrient supply and the foetal waste removal between the foetus and the mother. It starts to develop on the 7th day of fertilisation in the form of syncytio-trophoblasts projecting and invading the endometrial epithelium and gains its full thickness on the 4th month of pregnancy. Any insufficient placental development can lead to abnormal fetal growth and poor survival.

A normal placenta is responsible for the synthesis of glycogen, fatty acids, cholesterol, ammonia and lactate. It allows the transfer of the maternal antibodies, in the smallest form of immunoglobulin G (IgG), but blocks out some of the bacteria from reaching the foetus. It also protects the foetus from rejecting by the mother. In addition, it carries an important role of synthesising and secreting of a number of hormones, e.g. human chorionic gonadotrophin (hCG), human placental lactogen (hPL), progesterone and estrogen. These hormones help in the maternal physiological adaptation to support and maintain pregnancy, promote foetal growth and stimulate other hormone production, e.g. the foetal adrenal glucocorticoids and mineralcorticoids (Blackburn, 2003).

Toxic effect of a xenobiotic can be brought to the foetus by impairing the function of the placenta or acting directly onto the foetus. Small lipophilic substances cross the placenta most efficiently; on the contrary, hydrophilic substances have a slower rate of placental transfer. Melamine was found to be non-cytotoxic to trophoblast-derived BeWo cells (Partanen, 2012). *In vivo* placental transfer was demonstrated in near-term pregnant rats (Chu et al, 2010; Chan et al, 2011; Chu et al, 2013), also in rats at mid-pregnancy (Chu et al, 2013).

Transfer of melamine through the human term placenta can be detected in 5 min and in a dose-dependent manner, not involving the efflux ATP-binding cassette (ABC) transporters. Around 40% of the melamine added in the placental perfusion experiment passed through the placenta but no microscopic crystals, significant oedema or syncytiotrophoblastic vacuolisation was found (Partanen et al, 2012). These studies suggested the melamine diffuses through the placenta passively and its foetal toxicity can be due to the direct toxic effect onto the foetus itself.

Perfusing human term placentae was found to trigger a 50% decline of hCG production while placental alkaline phosphatase (PLAP) production increased, which can raise the risk of spontaneous start of labour and placental tissue damage brought by melamine (Partanen et al, 2012; Edelstam et al, 2007). This crystal-free but damaged placenta by a contact of melamine may thus allow easier diffusion of melamine across the barrier throughout pregnancy. At the same time, hCG can also stimulate the production of testosterone and corticosteroid by the foetal testes and adrenal gland and the production of progesterone by the placenta, suppress the maternal lymphocyte response for rejection of the placenta by the mother (Blackburn, 2003), thus a decrease in hCG level in earlier period of pregnancy may lead to impairment offoetal reproductive tract differentiation, lung maturation and foetal growth, etc. Moreover, the damaged placenta may provide a less favourable environment for the foetal growth which may lead to an intrauterine programming to a poor outcome in later life through epigenetic modifications (Lewis et al, 2011). Glucose transporters (GLUTs) are expressed on the placenta facilitating the glucose movement from the mother towards the placenta (Illsley, 2000), as a major energy source for the foetus. The placentally secreted hPL further helps the foetus to draw more glucose and amino acids from the maternal circulation. Besides, the placenta is also metabolically active, producing lactate, ketone bodies and ammonia as the alternative energy, glycogen synthesis and nitrogen sources, hence stimulating the foetal liver metabolism (Hay, 1994; Blackburn, 2003). Uteroplacental insufficiency may thus post a negative impact on the foetal nutritional status and impair liver growth, e.g. hepatic energy metabolism (Lane et al, 1996), hepatic mitochondrial redox states (Ogata et al, 1990) and glucose transport (Lane et al, 1999).

4.2. Melamine Distribution in Foetus and Neotates

Distribution of xenobiotic depends very much on the physiological factors. Placental transfer of xenobiotics can be influenced by the different stages of the placental development (Mihaly & Morgan, 1983). Similar to the changing physiology during the course of pregnancy, developing foetuses and neonates are experiencing rapid and tremendous modifications so as to adapt to the needs in different periods of growth. As a consequence, xenobiotics can show temporal changes of differential distribution from the developing foetuses to the infants. Toxicokinetic investigation showed melamine was distributed in liver the most, followed by brain and kidney in near-term rat foetuses. The maximum concentration of melamine was detected in the foetal liver and heart while melamine was distributed to and removed from the foetal brain and kidney comparatively slowly. The situation changed greatly 2 weeks after the birth of the rats. The proportion of melamine distributed to the developing kidney increased immensely after birth and to the brain in the opposite fashion. Distribution to the neonatal liver, lung, heart and spleen became comparable and much less than that of the kidney. Melamine in the neonatal kidney built up slowly with the maximum concentration 5 times of those of the other organs evaluated (Chu et al, 2013). Considering the fact that rat is born in a less developed state when compared with the human neonate, the rat kidney at 2 weeks after birth is comparable to the last trimester of the human foetal kidney (Tufro-McReddie et al, 1995). This 2-week-old rat kidney model can be a good estimation method for the effect of the xenobiotics on the development of the late human foetal kidney. An *in vivo* study using adult rat revealed the distribution of melamine in different brain region was not uniform: the mostly affected regions were hippocampus, cerebellum and striatum (Wu et al, 2009a). This implies that melamine can post different threats in the developing foetuses and infants in different stages of life. Clinical follow-up of the systems other than the urinary excretory system may be necessary if there is an *in utero* contact of the adulterant.

Since toxicokinetic study showed that foetal kidney, liver and brain were the organs with the highest melamine distributed (Chu et al, 2013) and skeletal malformation was also reported in another article (Kim et al, 2011), we would like to focus the discussion in these 4 developing organs.

4.3. Foetal Kidney and Pathology

Development of human foetal kidney starts at about the 4th week of gestation. Pronephroi (rudimentary and non-functional) and mesonephroi (developed and functional in early foetal stage) appear and pronephroi degenerate shortly. In week 5, metanephric blastema develops from the intermediate mesoderm and joins with the elongated ureteric bud; in week 6, renal tubules form by repeating branching and twisting of metanephric tubule, which will later form the functional nephrons. By week 9, the foetal kidneys begin to function and produce urine, although foetal wastes are still removed through the exchange between the foetal and the maternal circulation. By week 27, the mesonephroi will degenerate. The number of glomeruli increases gradually from 10th to 18th week and rapidly till 32nd week. Maturation and hypertrophy carry on in human infants until the 5 months after birth (Moore et al, 2013). Injury to the developing kidney prenatally as well as in early infancy can cause impairment of renal function in later life.

In the womb, foetus is surrounded by and suspending in a closed system of the amniotic fluid. Unlike the born child, the urine produced by the functional foetal kidney cannot remove waste at all. Instead, the waste excreted will be swallowed back by the foetus. Looping in this cycle, melamine may concentrate in the foetal kidney, resulting in a higher and higher chance of crystallisation. Moreover, the foetal renal blood flow is 3% of the cardiac output, only 1/8 of that of the adult. Towards term, renal tubules become longer and better developed while the urine flow is still low. Crystals can be easier to grow due to the foetal kidney's lower ability of flushing out the crystals formed in the delicate renal tubules.

There is no clinical report so far on the effect of *in utero* contact of melamine. The vast majority is the studies relating the intake of the contaminated infant formulae and the disease severity. The most common clinical presentation of the melamine-affected infant was AKI, nephrolithiasis and urolithiasis (Shang et al, 2012; Shi et al, 2012; Sun et al, 2009; Chen et al, 2010; Zhang et al, 2009; Wang et al, 2009). Infantile AKI episode is positively correlated to the development of chronic renal disease in later life (Mammen et al, 2012) and presumably relates to the increase in cardiovascular risk (Gansevoort et al, 2013).

Impaired renal development *in utero* can also lead to complications in later life. The weight and the relative weight of the kidney was once regarded as a standard for estimating the renal growth of a foetus however its large biological variation among individuals. To rule out the possible hypo- and hyperplasia affecting the kidney weight, 'medullary ray glomerular counting' has been introduced to replace the old method. The advantage of this method is that it takes the actively growing number of glomeruli under microscope as the criterion to assess the renal growth (Hinchliffe et al, 1992). Different developmental stages of the glomeruli can also be studied. An advanced maturity of the developing glomeruli was noticed in near-term rat foetuses in repeated dose of melamine relative to the control (Chu et al, unpublished data). Low nephron endowment at birth is associated with hypertension in adult life (Bagby, 2007) while high nephron endowment can be protective against hypertension (Walker et al, 2012). Therefore the advanced maturity of the melamine-affected foetal kidneys may be a response of triggering the rescue mechanism against the damage. The nephron number is inversely correlated to the mean glomerular volume, and perhaps also to the single nephron GFR. Renal developmental impairment is associated with cardiovascular dysfunction (Moritz et al, 2009). The long-term effect of the foetal nephrotoxicity of melamine should not be overlooked.

4.4. Foetal Liver and Pathology

In human, the foetal liver develops from the hepatic diverticulum in week 4 of an embryo. In week 5, the rapidly proliferating endodermal cells develop into the interlacing cords of hepatocytes, while the hepatic sinusoids first appear as the result of anastomosis of the hepatic cords. The foetal liver begins to make blood cells from the 6th week and bile from the 12th week. Similar to kidney, maturity of liver is not complete by the time of birth, but continues for 2 more years of life, and still exhibit the plasticity 12 months after birth (Moore et al, 2013). The foetal circulation brings about half of the oxygenated and nutrient-rich blood delivered by the umbilical vein to the foetal liver; the other portion is shunted off by the ductus venosus and diverted to other vital organs, e.g. brain (Moore et al, 2013).

Liver abnormalities including hepatomegaly, elevated aspartate amino-transferasemia, gallstone, liver lesions (Zhang et al, 2009), gradual progressive jaundice, abdominal distention, hepatic intumesce and bilirubin abnormality (Hu et al, 2012) were observed in infants taking melamine-laced formulae. These clinical evidences reveal the hepatotoxicity of melamine, which has not been the focus of the majority of the investigations. The foetal liver is responsible for lipid synthesis and haematopoiesis. Impairment of liver function during foetal development may perturb the lipid metabolism and fat deposition. Fatty liver is one of the most common respond to hepatic toxicity. Paediatric non-alcoholic fatty liver disease may increase the risk for cardiovascular disease in later life (Pacifico et al, 2011). Melamine-cyanuric acid crystals, but not the 2 compounds separately, are able to cause aggregation of human erythrocytes, haemolysis and rapid leakage of K^+, resulting from the pore formation in the erythrocyte membranes (Wang et al, 2010). Melamine alone can also inhibit some haem peroxidases, namely horseradish peroxidase, lactoperoxidase and cyclooxygenase-1 (Vanachayangkul & Tolleson, 2012). As a result, prenatal melamine contact may impair haematopoiesis, hostdefense mechanism and production of prostaglandins. Rapid growth of the foetus may also be retarded by the contact of melamine since foetal liver also actively produces insulin-like growth factors (IGFs) to stimulate cell proliferation, differentiation and metabolism (Gluckman, 1997).

4.5. Foetal Brain and Pathology

Brain and nervous system development is a more complicated process. It starts from the very beginning of the embryo development. At the 3rd week of gestation the neural plate and neural groove on the posterior appear by the overlying of ectoderm, which is induced by the notochord and paraxial mesenchyme. The neural plate and the neural tube form and the rostral and the caudal neuropores close in the 4th week. This marks the establishment of the vascular circulation for the neural tube. Thickening of the lateral walls of the neural tube and the diminishing in size of the neural canal at weeks 9 – 10 make the spinal cord. The neuroepithelium in the ventricular zone differentiates into different neuronal cell types, e.g. neurons, astrocytes, oligodentrocytes andgliablasts. Microglia are derived from mesenchymal cells (Moore et al, 2013). By week 6 of gestation, different part of the brain can be distinguished, e.g. corpus striatum, thalamus, hypothalamus, cerebral peduncles, cerebellum, pons and medulla (Carlson, 2013). Cellular proliferation, selective apoptotic cell death and migration of cells in cerebellum take place in weeks 6 to 16. The developing brain has gained almost all the cells by week 24 and migration of cells continues until term. Organisation and maturation of the cerebral cortex, formation of synapses and the internal granular layer in cerebellum will not finish until the 3rd trimester. Disturbance in the brain development during different periods by the differential distribution of melamine in brain parts will result in different corresponding disorders (Donkelaar et al, 2006).

Clinical description on the neurotoxicity of melamine is lacking, so as study using pregnant or neonatal animals. With the evidence of high distribution of melamine in the foetal brain, *in vitro* and animal behavioural experiments may have deciphered the risk behind. Impairment of spatial learning and memory associated with melamine intake was proven by the poor performance of water maze test by the infant rats: decreasing in time spent in the target quadrant and increasing in escape latency (An et al, 2012; Yang et al, 2011). The hyperpolarisation of neurons was altered. The melamine-induced decrease in the frequencies of the spontaneous and the minitura excitatory postsynaptic currents inhibited the presynaptic glutamate transmission of the primary rat hippocampal neuron culture (Yang et al, 2011). Melamine induced a shift towards hyperpolarisation of neurons, increased spontaneous firing and enhanced excitability of the rat hippocampus pyrimadal neurons, which implied a possibility of damage to the central nervous system of the pre-school children (Yang et al, 2010). Melamine can decrease the basal synaptic transmission in the hippocampal slices due to the reduction of presynaptic function. Long-term potentiation was impaired but not the long-term depression in young neonates as well as in adolescence. Performance of water maze test also worsened, without affecting the locomotor activity in the open field test (Yang et al, 2012). Neonatal rats were more sensitive to the neurotoxicity of melamine and they became less susceptible with increase in age. Oxidative stress and increased in neuronal apoptosis were also resulted in melamine exposure. Activities of superoxide dismutase (SOD) and capspase-3 decreased and Ca^{2+} level increased, shrinkage of hippocampal neurons and chromatin congregation were also reported (Han et al, 2011; Wang et al, 2011). *In vivo* evidences also showed increased superoxide anion radical, hydroxyl free radical and malondialdehyde, decrease in activities of SOD and GSH-peroxidase and decrease in adenosine-triphosphatein melamine-administered rat hippocampus (An et al, 2012). Microscopic observation of the effect of melamine on whole embryo culture revealed open neural tube and atrioventricular defects induced by the compound with the retarded embryo growth. This suggests the brain damage by melamine can start at very early in the womb (Chu et al, unpublished data).

4.6. Foetal Skeletal Development and Pathology

Skeletal development starts with the appearance of somites from the 3rd week of pregnancy. The sclerotome on the ventromedial side later forms the vertebratae and ribs while the dorsolateral dermomyotome comprises the myotome and dermatome, which will result in muscle and skin. Towards the end of week 4, the sclerotome forms a loose structure of mesenchyme which later condenses. Flat bones are formed in membranous shealths and ossified in the process called membranous bone formation. The limb bones are developed from mesenchymes ossification of cartilage bones from the 5th week, which is named as endochondral bone formation (Moore et al, 2013). Detailed description of effect of melamine of *in utero* contact was given in a rat experiment. The authors reported enlarged fontanel, incomplete ossification of supraoccipotalis, incomplete ossification of interparietal, bipartite ossification of sternebra and incomplete ossification of pubis were observed together with lower body weight. A decrease in the number of the ossification centres of all four limbs and the sacral and the caudal vertebra were also observed. This indicated melamine delayed the skeletal development and probably the overall growth of the foetus (Kim et al, 2011).

5. Mechanistic Studies

Mechanistic studies have been carried out only in adult animals. These pieces of information have tried to decipher the melamine toxicity in molecular level, e.g. recruitment of immune cells (Umekawa et al, 2003; Hsieh et al, 2012; Lu et al, 2012; Liu et al, 2012), repair and regeneration of renal tubules and restoration of kidney function after injury (Camacho et al, 2011; Zhang et al, 2012; Early et al, 2013), formation of stones, association with cytoskeleton, cell fraction-related to apoptosis and necrosis (Liu et al, 2012). Metabolism disturbances were also revealed: inflammation-induced up-regulation of the kynurenine pathway of the tryptophan metabolism, involvement of the urea cycle-related polyamine metabolism in impairment of renal function (Xie et al, 2010), inhibition of tricarboxylic acid cycle and increase in anaerobic cell respiration (Xie et al, 2010; Sun et al, 2012; Kim et al, 2012; Ma et al, 2011), metabolism of carbohydrates, lipids as well as proteins (Sun et al, 2012), and metabolisms of GSH, arginine and proline (Ma et al, 2011). Nevertheless, the development of the various metabolisms described above in foetus is not completely known and whether or not these information can predict the *in utero* toxicity of melamine. Melamine can also interact with DNA (Shen et al, 2011); however, the product of this interaction is not yet known. Although there is no evidence of melamine causing tumours in foetal and neonatal animals as far as reported, we cannot ignore its carcinogenic properties learnt from the experiments done as early as in the 1980s (Melnick et al, 1984; Ogasawara et al, 1995).

Conclusion

In order to correctly access the risk of ingesting melamine in different stage of life, detailed characterisation of the toxic effects, accumulative effects, distribution of the contaminant, amount and frequency of intake of the contaminant, the concentration of the contaminant detected in daily food and the ever-changing physiological conditions throughout life have to be taken into account.

Toxic substances are given a reference safety level for oral ingestion by the Codex Alimentarius Committee, which is known as the tolerable daily intake (TDI). However, if a chemical is carcinogenic, no threshold level is applicable. Since the 2008 scandal, the TDI of melamine is revised and lowered to 0.2 ppm/day for both infants and adults (Ingelfinger, 2008). The maximum level of melamine in general food and animal feed is then set as 2.5 mg/kg and a lower allowance is given to the liquid infant milk and the powdered infant formulae as 0.15 and 1 mg/kg, respectively (WHO, 2012).

Differential distribution of a xenobiotic and the sensitivity of the developing organs make the prediction of its toxicity difficult. Alteration of macromolecule metabolism, delay in foetal growth and any epigenetic changes brought by the *in utero* contact of melamine can lead to developmental programming, which in turn will lead to health problems in the later life. Longer clinical follow-up or longitudinal animal study involving F1 generation may be insightful in giving more information in the long-term influence of the contaminant.

ACKNOWLEDGMENT

This study was supported by a funding on Studies Related to Melamine Incident from Food and Health Bureau, Hong Kong Special Administration Region (MI-BS-06).

REFERENCES

An L, Li Z, Yang Z, Zhang T. (2012). Melamine induced cognitive impairment associated with oxidative damage in rat's hippocampus. *Pharmacol. Biochem. Behav.*, 102(2):196-202.

Bagby SP. (2007). Maternal nutrition, low nephron number, and hypertension in later life: pathways of nutritional programming. *J. Nutr.*, 137(4):1066-72.

Barboza D. (2008, Nov 13). *Hong Kong finds tainted Chinese fish feed.* Retrieved Aug 20, 2013, from The New York Times: http://www.nytimes.com/2008/11/13/world/asia/13china.html.

Barboza D, Barrionuevo A. (2007, April 30). *Filler in Animal Feed Is Open Secret in China.* Retrieved Aug 19, 2013, from The New York Times: http://www.nytimes.com/2007/04/30/business/worldbusiness/30food.html?pagewanted=all.

Baynes RE, Barlow B, Mason SE, Riviere JE. (2010). Disposition of melamine residues in blood and milk from dairy goats exposed to an oral bolus of melamine. *Food Chem. Toxicol.*, 48(8-9):2542-6.

Baynes RE, Smith G, Mason SE, Barrett E, Barlow BM, Riviere JE. (2008). Pharmacokinetics of melamine in pigs following intravenous administration. *Food Chem. Toxicol.*, 46(3):1196-200.

BBC News. (2010, Feb 8). *China searches for 100 tonnes of melamine-tainted milk.* Retrieved Aug 20, 2013, from BBC News: http://news.bbc.co.uk/2/hi/asia-pacific/8503576.stm.

Blackburn ST. (2003). *Maternal, fetal, & neonatal physiology : a clinical perspective, 2nd ed.* St. Louis, MO: Saunders.

Bradley EL, Boughtflower V, Smith TL, Speck DR, Castle L. (2005). Survey of the migration of melamine and formaldehyde from melamine food contact articles available on the UK market. *Food Addit. Contam.*, 22(6):597-606.

Bradley EL, Castle L, Day JS, Ebner I, Ehlert K, Helling R, Koster S, Leak J, Pfaff K. (2010). Comparison of the migration of melamine from melamine-formaldehyde plastics ('melaware') into various food simulants and foods themselves. *Food Addit. Contam. Part A Chem. Anal. Control. Expo Risk Assess*, 27(12):1755-64.

Brown CA, Jeong KS, Poppenga RH, Puschner B, Miller DM, Ellis AE, Kang KI, Sum S, Cistola AM, Brown SA. (2007). Outbreaks of renal failure associated with melamine and cyanuric acid in dogs and cats in 2004 and 2007. *J. Vet. Diagn. Invest.*, 19(5):525-31.

Buur JL, Baynes RE, Riviere JE. (2008). Estimating meat withdrawal times in pigs exposed to melamine contaminated feed using a physiologically based pharmacokinetic model. *Regul. Toxicol. Pharmacol.*, 51(3):324-31.

Camacho L, Kelly KP, Beland FA, Gamboa da Costa G. (2011). Gene expression of biomarkers of nephrotoxicity in F344 rats co-exposed to melamine and cyanuric acid for seven days. *Toxicol Lett.*, 206(2):166-71.

Carlson B. (2013). *Human Embryology and Developmental Biology.* Saunders.

CFS HK. (2009, Apr 30). Centre for Food Safety, Hong Kong.*Unsatisfactory results of testing of Melamine in Food Samples.* Retrieved Aug 20, 2013, from CFS HK: http://www.cfs.gov.hk/cgi-bin/cfsnew/melamine/unsat_ecsvread.pl.

CFS HK. (2010, Nov). Centre for Food Safety, Hong Kong.*Safety of melamine-ware available for use on local food premises.* Retrieved Aug 20, 2013, from CFS HK: http://www.cfs.gov.hk/english/programme/programme_rafs/files/RA_Study_on_Melamine-ware_Final_Report_Nov 2010_e.pdf.

Chan JY, Lau CM, Ting TL, Mak TC, Chan MH, Lam CW, Ho CS, Wang CC, Fok TF, Fung KP. (2011). Gestational and lactational transfer of melamine following gavage administration of a single dose to rats. *Food Chem. Toxicol.*, 49(7):1544-8.

Chen WC, Wu SY, Liu HP, Chang CH, Chen HY, Chen HY, Tsai CH, Chang YC, Tsai FJ, Man KM, Liu PL, Lin FY, Shen JL, Lin WY, Chen YH. (2010). Identification of melamine/cyanuric acid-containing nephrolithiasis by infrared spectroscopy. *J. Clin. Lab. Anal.*, 24(2):92-9.

Cheng G, Shapir N, Sadowsky MJ, Wackett LP. (2005). Allophanate hydrolase, not urease, functions in bacterial cyanuric acid metabolism. *Appl. Environ. Microbiol.*, 71(8):4437-45.

Chik Z, Haron DE, Ahmad ED, Taha H, Mustafa AM. (2011). Analysis of melamine migration from melamine food contact articles. *Food Addit. Contam. Part A Chem. Anal. Control. Expo Risk Assess*, 28(7):967-73.

Chu CY, Chu KO, Chan JY, Liu XZ, Ho CS, Wong CK, Lau CM, Ting TL, Fok TF, Fung KP, Wang CC. (2010). Distribution of melamine in rat foetuses and neonates. *Toxicol. Lett.*, 199(3):398-402.

Chu CY, Chu KO, Ho CS, Kwok SS, Chan HM, Fung KP, Wang CC. (2013). Melamine in prenatal and postnatal organs in rats. *Reprod. Toxicol.*, 35:40-7.

Cianciolo RE, Bischoff K, Ebel JG, Van Winkle TJ, Goldstein RE, Serfilippi LM. (2008). Clinicopathologic, histologic, and toxicologic findings in 70 cats inadvertently exposed to pet food contaminated with melamine and cyanuric acid. *J. Am. Vet. Med. Assoc.*, 233(5):729-3.

Cocchi M, Vascellari M, Gallina A, Agnoletti F, Angeletti R, Mutinelli F. (2010). Canine nephrotoxicosis induced by melamine-contaminated pet food in Italy. *J. Vet. Med. Sci.*,72(1):103-7.

Codex Alimentarius Commission. (2011). *CODEX STAN 72 – 1981.* Retrieved Aug 20, 2013, from Codex Alimentarius: http://www.codexalimentarius.org/download/standards/288/CXS_072e.pdf.

Conlan S, Kong HH, Segre JA. (2012). Species-level analysis of DNA sequence data from the NIH Human Microbiome Project. *PLoS One*, 7(10):e47075. doi: 10.1371/journal.pone.0047075.

Cruywagen CW, Stander MA, Adonis M, Calitz T. (2009). Hot topic: pathway confirmed for the transmission of melamine from feed to cow's milk. *J. Dairy Sci.*, 92(5):2046-50.

Dai ZL, Li XL, Xi PB, Zhang J, Wu G, Zhu WY. (2012). Metabolism of select amino acids in bacteria from the pig small intestine. *Amino Acids*, 42(5):1597-608.

Dakin, HD, Dudley, HW. (1914). Some limitations of the Kjeldahl method. *J. Biol. Chem.*, 275-80.

Dodge AG, Wackett LP, Sadowsky MJ. (2012). Plasmid localization and organization of melamine degradation genes in Rhodococcus sp. strain Mel. *Appl. Environ. Microbiol.*, 78(5):1397-403.

Donkelaar HJ, Lammens M, & Hori A. (2006). *Clinical Neuroembryology : Development and Developmental Disorders of the Human Central Nervous System.* Berlin, Heidelberg: Springer-Verlag Berlin Heidelberg.

Duong A, Steinmaus C, McHale CM, Vaughan CP, Zhang L. (2011). Reproductive and developmental toxicity of formaldehyde: a systematic review. *Mutat. Res.*, 728(3):118-38.

Early RJ, Yu H, Mu XP, Xu H, Guo L, Kong Q, Zhou J, He B, Yang X, Huang H, Hu E, Jiang Y. (2013). Repeat oral dose toxicity studies of melamine in rats and monkeys. *Arch. Toxicol.*, 87(3):517-27.

Eaton RW, Karns JS. (1991). Cloning and analysis of s-triazine catabolic genes from Pseudomonas sp. strain NRRLB-12227. *J. Bacteriol.*, 173(3): 1215-22.

Edelstam G, Karlsson C, Westgren M, Löwbeer C, Swahn ML. (2007). Human chorionic gonadatropin (hCG) during third trimester pregnancy. *Scand. J. Clin. Lab. Invest.*, 67(5):519-25.

EFSA. (2008, Sep 24). European Food Safety Authority. Statement of EFSA on risks for public health due to the presences of melamine in infant milk and other milk products in China. Retrieved Aug 20, 2013, from *The EFSA Journal:* http://www.efsa.europa.eu/en/efsajournal/doc/807.pdf.

El-Sayed WS, El-Baz AF, & Othman AM. (2006). Biodegradation of melamine formaldehyde by Micrococcus sp. strain MF-1 isolated from aminoplastic wastewater effluent. *Int. Biodeterior. Biodegrad.*, 57(2):75–81.

Erickson LE, Lee KH. (1989). Degradation of atrazine and related s-triazines. *Crit. Rev. Environ. Control*, 19:1-14.

European Chemical News. (2004). *Product Profile: Melamine, July 26, 2004. European Chemical News*. Retrieved 8 5, 2013, from ICIS.com: http://www.icis.com/Articles/2004/07/23/598783/product+profile+melamine.html.

Gansevoort RT, Correa-Rotter R, Hemmelgarn BR, Jafar TH, Heerspink HJ, Mann JF, Matsushita K, Wen CP. (2013). Chronic kidney disease and cardiovascular risk: epidemiology, mechanisms, and prevention. *Lancet*, 382(9889):339-52.

Gao CQ, Wu SG, Yue HY, Ji F, Zhang HJ, Liu QS, Fan ZY, Liu FZ, Qi GH. (2010). Toxicity of dietary melamine to laying ducks: biochemical and histopathological changes and residue in eggs. *J. Agric. Food Chem.*, 58(8):5199-205.

Gei AF, Hankins GD. (2001). Cardiac disease and pregnancy. *Obstet. Gynecol. Clin. North Am.*, 28(3):465-512.

Gluckman PD. (1997). Endocrine and nutritional regulation of prenatal growth. *Acta Paediatr. Suppl.*, 423:153-7.

Goldman A, Lee D. (2007, May 4). *Reported pet deaths at 8,500, FDA says.* Retrieved Aug 19, 2013, from Los Angeles Times: http://articles.latimes.com/2007/may/04/business/fi-petfood4.

González J, Puschner B, Pérez V, Ferreras MC, Delgado L, Muñoz M, Pérez C, Reyes LE, Velasco J, Fernández V, García-Marín JF. (2009). Nephrotoxicosis in Iberian piglets subsequent to exposure to melamine and derivatives in Spain between 2003 and 2006. *J. Vet. Diagn. Invest.*, 21(4):558-63.

Goodman B. (2007, Mar 30). *F.D.A. Tests Show Chemical in Pet Food.* Retrieved Aug 19, 2013, from The New York Times: http://www.nytimes.com/2007/03/30/us/30cnd-pet.html.

Han YG, Liu SC, Zhang T, Yang Z. (2011). Induction of apoptosis by melamine in differentiated PC12 cells. *Cell Mol. Neurobiol.*, 31(1):65-71.

Hapeman CJ, Karns JS, Shelton DR. (1995). Total mineralization of aqueous atrazine in the presence of ammonium nitrate using ozone and Klebsiella terragena (strain drs-i): mechanistic considerations for pilot scale disposal. *J. Agric. Food Chem.*, 43(5):1383–91.

Hay WJ. (1994). Placental transport of nutrients to the fetus. *Horm. Res.*, 42(4-5):215-22.

Heikkilä A, Erkkola R. (1994). Review of beta-lactam antibiotics in pregnancy. The need for adjustment of dosage schedules. *Clin. Pharmacokinet.*, 27(1):49-62.

Hinchliffe SA, Sargent PH, Chan YF, van Velzen D, Howard CV, Hutton JL, Rushton DI. (1992). "Medullary ray glomerular counting" as a method of assessment of human nephrogenesis. *Pathol. Res. Pract.*, 188(6):775-82.

Hsieh TJ, Hsieh PC, Tsai YH, Wu CF, Liu CC, Lin MY, Wu MT. (2012). Melamine induces human renal proximal tubular cell injury via transforming growth factor-β and oxidative stress. *Toxicol. Sci.*, 130(1):17-32.

Hu P, Lu L, Hu B, Zhang CR. (2010). The size of melamine-induced stones is dependent on the melamine content of the formula fed, but not on duration of exposure. *Pediatr. Nephrol.*, 25(3):565-6.

Hu P, Wang J, Zhang M, Hu B, Lu L, Zhang CR, Du PF. (2012). Liver involvement in melamine-associated nephrolithiasis. *Arch. Iran Med.*, 15(4):247-8.

Illsley NP. (2000). Placental glucose transport in diabetic pregnancy. *Clin. Obstet. Gynecol.*, 43(1):116-26.

Ingelfinger JR. (2008). Melamine and the global implications of food contamination. *N. Engl. J. Med.*, 359(26):2745-8.

Jacob CC, Von Tungeln LS, Vanlandingham M, Beland FA, Gamboa da Costa G. (2012). Pharmacokinetics of melamine and cyanuric acid and their combinations in F344 rats. *Toxicol. Sci.*, 126(2):317-24.

Jang YH, Hwang S, Chang SB, Ku J, Chung DS. (2009). Acid dissociation constants of melamine derivatives from density functional theory calculations. *J. Phys. Chem. A*, 113(46):13036-40.

Jeong WI, Do SH, Jeong da H, Chung JY, Yang HJ, Yuan DW, Hong IH, Park JK, Goo MJ, Jeong KS. (2006). Canine renal failure syndrome in three dogs. *J. Vet. Sci.*, 7(3):299-301.

Jian X, Raina P. (2011, Jul 19). *Chinese Pigs Fed Poisoned Milk Powder* . Retrieved Aug 20, 2013, from The Epoch Times: http://www. Theepoch times.com/n2/china-news/chinese-pigs-fed-poisoned-milk-powder-59286.html.

Jingbin W, Ndong M, Kai H, Matsuno K, Kayama F. (2010). Placental transfer of melamine and its effects on rat dams and fetuses. *Food Chem. Toxicol.*, 48(7):1791-5.

Jutzi K, Cook AM, Hütter R. (1982). The degradative pathway of the s-triazine melamine. The steps to ring cleavage. *Biochem. J.*, 208(3):679-84.

Kim SH, Lee IC, Lim JH, Shin IS, Moon C, Kim SH, Park SC, Kim HC, Kim JC. (2011). Effects of melamine on pregnant dams and embryo-fetal development in rats. *J. Appl. Toxicol.*, 31(6):506-14.

Kim TH, Ahn MY, Lim HJ, Lee YJ, Shin YJ, De U, Lee J, Lee BM, Kim S, Kim HS. (2012). Evaluation of metabolomic profiling against renal toxicity in Sprague-Dawley rats treated with melamine and cyanuric acid. *Arch. Toxicol.*, 86(12):1885-97.

Kinoshita H. (1953). Synthesis of melamine from urea, I. *Rev. Phys. Chem. Jpn.*, 1-9.

Kinoshita H. (1954). Synthesis of melamine from urea, II. *Rev. Phys. Chem. Jpn.*, 19-27.

Kontchou CY, Gschwind N. (1999). Biodegradation of s-triazine compounds by a stable mixed bacterial community. *Ecotoxicol. Environ. Saf.*, 43(1):47-56.

Krauer B, Dayer P, Anner R. (1984). Changes in serum albumin and alpha 1-acid glycoprotein concentrations during pregnancy: an analysis of fetal-maternal pairs. *Br. J. Obstet. Gynaecol.*, 91(9):875-81.

Lam HS, Ng PC, Chu WC, Wong W, Chan DF, Ho SS, Wong KT, Ahuja AT, Li CK. (2008). Renal screening in children after exposure to low dose melamine in Hong Kong: cross sectional study. *BMJ*, 337:a2991.

Lane RH, Crawford SE, Flozak AS, Simmons RA. (1999). Localization and quantification of glucose transporters in liver of growth-retarded fetal and neonatal rats. *Am. J. Physiol.*, 276(1 Pt 1):E135-42.

Lane RH, Flozak AS, Ogata ES, Bell GI, Simmons RA. (1996). Altered hepatic gene expression of enzymes involved in energy metabolism in the growth-retarded fetal rat. *Pediatr. Res.*, 39(3):390-4.

Lash LH. (1994). Role of renal metabolism in risk to toxic chemicals. *Environ. Health Perspect.*, 102 Suppl 11:75-9.

Lewis RM, Cleal JK, Godfrey KM. (2011). The placental role in fetal programming. In R. Gupta, *Reproductive and developmental toxicology* (pp. 1039-50). Amsterdam; Boston: Elsevier.

Lim LO, Scherer SJ, Shuler KD, Toth JP. (1990). Disposition of Cyromazine in Plants under Environmental Conditions. *J. Agric. Food Chem.*, 38(3): 860-4.

Liu JD, Liu JJ, Yuan JH, Tao GH, Wu DS, Yang XF, Yang LQ, Huang HY, Zhou L, Xu XY, Hu JJ, Zhuang ZX. (2012). Proteome of melamine urinary bladder stones and implication for stone formation. *Toxicol. Lett.*, 212(3):307-14.

Lü MB, Yan L, Guo JY, Li Y, Li GP, Ravindran V. (2009). Melamine residues in tissues of broilers fed diets containing graded levels of melamine. *Poult. Sci.*, 88(10):2167-70.

Lu X, Gao B, Wang Y, Liu Z, Yasui T, Liu P, Liu J, Emmanuel N, Zhu Q, Xiao C. (2012). Renal tubular epithelial cell injury, apoptosis and inflammation are involved in melamine-related kidney stone formation. *Urol. Res.*, 40(6):717-23.

Lu X, Wang J, Cao X, Li M, Xiao C, Yasui T, Gao B. (2011). Gender and urinary pH affect melamine-associated kidney stone formation risk. *Urol. Ann.*, 3(2):71-4.

Lund KH, Petersen JH. (2006). Migration of formaldehyde and melamine monomers from kitchen- and tableware made of melamine plastic. *Food Addit. Contam.*, 23(9):948-55.

Ma C, Kang H, Liu Q, Zhu R, Cao Z. (2011). Insight into potential toxicity mechanisms of melamine: an in silico study. *Toxicology*, 283(2-3):96-100.

Mammen C, Al Abbas A, Skippen P, Nadel H, Levine D, Collet JP, Matsell DG. (2012). Long-term risk of CKD in children surviving episodes of acute kidney injury in the intensive care unit: a prospective cohort study. *Am. J. Kidney Dis.*, 59(4):523-30.

Mast RW, Jeffcoat AR, Sadler BM, Kraska RC, Friedman MA. (1983). Metabolism, disposition and excretion of [14C]melamine in male Fischer 344 rats. *Food Chem. Toxicol.*, 21(6):807-10.

Mattison DR, Blann E, Malek A. (1991). Physiological alterations during pregnancy: impact on toxicokinetics. *Fundam. Appl. Toxicol.*, 16(2):215-8.

Melnick RL, Boorman GA, Haseman JK, Montali RJ, Huff J. (1984). Urolithiasis and bladder carcinogenicity of melamine in rodents. *Toxicol. Appl. Pharmacol.*, 72(2):292-303.

Mihaly GW, Morgan DJ. (1983). Placental drug transfer: effects of gestational age and species. *Pharmacol. Ther.*, 23(2):253-66.

Moore KL, Persaud TVN, Torchia MG. (2013). *The developing human: clinically oriented embryology, 9th ed.* Philadelphia, PA: Saunders/ Elsevier.

Moritz KM, Singh RR, Probyn ME, Denton KM. (2009). Developmental programming of a reduced nephron endowment: more than just a baby's birth weight. *Am. J. Physiol. Renal. Physiol.*, 296(1):F1-9.

Nilubol D, Pattanaseth T, Boonsri K, Pirarat N, Leepipatpiboon N. (2009). Melamine- and cyanuric acid-associated renal failure in pigs in Thailand. *Vet. Pathol.*, 46(6):1156-9.

Ogasawara H, Imaida K, Ishiwata H, Toyoda K, Kawanishi T, Uneyama C, Hayashi S, Takahashi M, Hayashi Y. (1995). Urinary bladder carcinogenesis induced by melamine in F344 male rats: correlation between carcinogenicity and urolith formation. *Carcinogenesis*, 16(11):2773-7.

Ogata ES, Swanson SL, Collins JW Jr, Finley SL. (1990). Intrauterine growth retardation: altered hepatic energy and redox states in the fetal rat. *Pediatr. Res.*, 27(1):56-63.

Pacifico L, Nobili V, Anania C, Verdecchia P, Chiesa C. (2011). Pediatric nonalcoholic fatty liver disease, metabolic syndrome and cardiovascular risk. *World J. Gastroenterol.*, 17(26):3082-91.

Panesar NS, Chan KW, Lo WS, Leung VH, Ho CS. (2010). Co-contamination, but not mammalian cell conversion of melamine to cyanuric acid the likely cause of melamine-cyanurate nephrolithiasis. *Clin. Chim. Acta*, 411(21-22):1830-1.

Pang J, Li GQ, Li CR, Yang XY, Lu X, Hu XX, Zhai QQ, Zhang WX, Jiang JD, You XF. (2013). Toxicokinetic study of melamine in the presence and absence of cyanuric acid in rats. *J. Appl. Toxicol.*, 33(6):444-50.

Partanen H, Vähäkangas K, Woo CS, Auriola S, Veid J, Chen Y, Myllynen P, El Nezami H. (2012). Transplacental transfer of melamine. *Placenta*, 33(1):60-6.

Patakioutas G, Savvas D, Matakoulis C, Sakellarides T, Albanis T. (2007). Application and fate of Cyromazine in a closed-cycle hydroponic cultivation of bean (Phaseolus vulgaris L.). *J. Agric. Food Chem.*, 55(24): 9928-35.

Rasmussen PE, Nielsen FR. (1988). Hydronephrosis during pregnancy: a literature survey. *Eur. J. Obstet. Gynecol. Reprod. Biol.*, 27(3):249-59.

Reimschuessel R, Evans E, Andersen WC, Turnipseed SB, Karbiwnyk CM, Mayer TD, Nochetto C, Rummel NG, Gieseker CM. (2010). Residue depletion of melamine and cyanuric acid in catfish and rainbow trout following oral administration. *J. Vet. Pharmacol. Ther.*, 33(2):172-82.

Root DS, Hongtrakul T, Dauterman WC. (1996). Studies on the Absorption, Residues and Metabolism of Cyromazine in Tomatoes. *Pesticide Science*, 48(1):25-30.

Rosenberg, E., Sergienko, R., Abu-Ghanem, S., Wiznitzer, A., Romanowsky, I., Neulander, E., & Sheiner, E. (2011). Nephrolithiasis during pregnancy: characteristics, complications, and pregnancy outcome. *World J. Urol.*, 29(6):743-7.

Seffernick JL, Dodge AG, Sadowsky MJ, Bumpus JA, Wackett LP. (2010). Bacterial ammeline metabolism via guanine deaminase. *J. Bacteriol.*, 192(4):1106-12.

Seffernick JL, Shapir N, Schoeb M, Johnson G, Sadowsky MJ, Wackett LP. (2002). Enzymatic degradation of chlorodiamino-s-triazine. *Appl. Environ. Microbiol.*, 68(9):4672-5.

Shang P, Chang H, Yue ZJ, Shi W, Zhang H, Tang X, He Q, Wang W. (2012). Acute kidney injury caused by consumption of melamine-contaminated infant formula in 47 children: a multi-institutional experience in diagnosis, treatment and follow-up. *Urol. Res.*, 40(4):293-8.

Shelton DR, Karns JS, McCarty GW, Durham DR. (1997). Metabolism of melamine by Klebsiella terragena. *Appl. Environ. Microbiol.*, 63(7): 2832-5.

Shen HY, Liu YQ, Gao J, Zhen HM, Zhu N, Li J. (2011). In vitro study of DNA interaction with melamine and its related compounds. *DNA Cell Biol.*, 30(4):255-64.

Shi GQ, Wang ZJ, Feng ZJ, Gao YJ, Di Liu J, Shen T, Li M, Yang J, Xu HB, Jiang XH, Wang ZN, Cai M, Wang YM, Zhu YF, Liu HH, Wang R, Xiong WY, Wang ZT, Yang WZ, Hou PS, Zeng G, Wang Y. (2012). A survey of urolithiasis in young children fed infant formula contaminated with melamine in two townships of Gansu, China. *Biomed. Environ. Sci.*, 25(2):149-55.

Stine, C., Nochetto, C., Evans, E., Gieseker, C., Mayer, T., Hasbrouck, N., & Reimschuessel, R. (2012). Depletion of melamine and cyanuric acid in serum from catfish Ictalurus punctatus and rainbow trout Onchorhynchus mykiss. *Food Chem. Toxicol.*, 50(10):3426-32.

Sugita T, Ishiwata H, Yoshihira K. (1990). Release of formaldehyde and melamine from tableware made of melamine-formaldehyde resin. *Food Addit. Contam.*, 7(1):21-7.

Sun N, Shen Y, Sun Q, Li XR, Jia LQ, Zhang GJ, Zhang WP, Chen Z, Fan JF, Jiang YP, Feng DC, Zhang RF, Zhu XY, Xiao HZ. (2009). Diagnosis and treatment of melamine-associated urinary calculus complicated with acute renal failure in infants and young children. *Chin. Med. J. (Engl)*, 122(3): 245-51.

Sun YJ, Wang HP, Liang YJ, Yang L, Li W, Wu YJ. (2012). An NMR-based metabonomic investigation of the subacute effects of melamine in rats. *J. Proteome Res.*, 11(4):2544-50.

Takagi K, Fujii K, Yamazaki K, Harada N, Iwasaki A. (2012). Biodegradation of melamine and its hydroxy derivatives by a bacterial consortium containing a novel Nocardioides species. *Appl. Microbiol. Biotechnol.*, 94(6):1647-56.

Tufro-McReddie A, Romano LM, Harris JM, Ferder L, Gomez RA. (1995). Angiotensin II regulates nephrogenesis and renal vascular development. *Am. J. Physiol.*, 269(1 Pt 2):F110-5.

Umekawa T, Chegini N, Khan SR. (2003). Increased expression of monocyte chemoattractant protein-1 (MCP-1) by renal epithelial cells in culture on exposure to calcium oxalate, phosphate and uric acid crystals. *Nephrol. Dial Transplant.*, 18(4):664-9.

Vanachayangkul P, Tolleson WH. (2012). Inhibition of heme peroxidases by melamine. *Enzyme Res.*, 416062, Epub 2012 Jul 18.

Wackett LP, Sadowsky MJ, Martinez B, Shapir N. (2002). Biodegradation of atrazine and related s-triazine compounds: from enzymes to field studies. *Appl. Microbiol. Biotechnol.*, 58(1):39-45.

Walker KA, Cai X, Caruana G, Thomas MC, Bertram JF, Kett MM. (2012). High nephron endowment protects against salt-induced hypertension. *Am. J. Physiol. Renal. Physiol.*, 303(2):F253-8.

Wang C, Qin X, Huang B, He F, Zeng C. (2010). Hemolysis of human erythrocytes induced by melamine-cyanurate complex. *Biochem. Biophys. Res. Commun.*, 402(4):773-7.

Wang IJ, Wu YN, Wu WC, Leonardi G, Sung YJ, Lin TJ, Wang CL, Kuo CF, Wu KY, Cheng WC, Chan CC, Chen PC, Lin SL. (2009). The association of clinical findings and exposure profiles with melamine associated nephrolithiasis. *Arch. Dis. Child*, 94(11):883-7.

Wang Y, Liu F, Wei Y, Liu D. (2011). The effect of exogenous melamine on rat hippocampal neurons. *Toxicol. Ind. Health*, 27(6):571-6.

WHO. (2009).World Health Organization.*Background paper on occurrence of melamine in foods and feed.* Retrieved Aug 20, 2013, from WHO.int: http://www.who.int/foodsafety/fs_management/Melamine_3.pdf.

WHO. (2012, Jul 4).World Health Organization.*UN strengthens regulations on melamine, seafood, melons, dried figs and labelling*. Retrieved from World Health Organization - Media centre: http://www.who.int/mediacentre/news/releases/2012/codex_20120704/en/index.html.

Wu YT, Huang CM, Lin CC, Ho WA, Lin LC, Chiu TF, Tarng DC, Lin CH, Tsai TH. (2009a). Determination of melamine in rat plasma, liver, kidney, spleen, bladder and brain by liquid chromatography-tandem mass spectrometry. *J. Chromatogr. A*, 1216(44):7595-601.

Wu YN, Zhao YF, Li JG; Melamine Analysis Group. (2009b). A survey on occurrence of melamine and its analogues in tainted infant formula in China. *Biomed. Environ. Sci.*, 22(2):95-9.

Xie G, Zheng X, Qi X, Cao Y, Chi Y, Su M, Ni Y, Qiu Y, Liu Y, Li H, Zhao A, Jia W. (2010). Metabonomic evaluation of melamine-induced acute renal toxicity in rats. *J. Proteome Res.*, 9(1):125-33.

Xinhua Net. (2007, Feb 27). *Chinese Premier asks entrepreneurs to be more ethical.* Retrieved Aug 20, 2013, from English.news.cn: http://news.xinhuanet.com/english2010/china/2010-02/27/c_13190700.htm.

Xinhua Net. (2008, Sep 12). *China starts probe into baby powder milk contamination as more cases reported.* Retrieved Aug 20, 2013, from Xinhua Net: http://news.xinhuanet.com/english/2008-09/12/content_9951527.htm.

Yang J, An L, Yao Y, Yang Z, Zhang T. (2011). Melamine impairs spatial cognition and hippocampal synaptic plasticity by presynaptic inhibition of glutamatergic transmission in infant rats. *Toxicology*, 289(2-3):167-74.

Yang JJ, Tian YT, Yang Z, Zhang T. (2010). Effect of melamine on potassium currents in rat hippocampal CA1 neurons. *Toxicol. In Vitro*, 24(2):397-403.

Yang Y, Xiong GJ, Yu DF, Cao J, Wang LP, Xu L, Mao RR.(2012). Acute low-dose melamine affects hippocampal synaptic plasticity and behavior in rats. *Toxicol. Lett.*, 214(1):63-8.

Yokley RA, Mayer LC, Rezaaiyan R, Manuli ME, Cheung MW. (2000). Analytical method for the determination of cyromazine and melamine residues in soil using LC-UV and GC-MSD. *J. Agric. Food Chem.*, 48(8): 3352-8.

Zhang L, Wu LL, Wang YP, Liu AM, Zou CC, Zhao ZY.. (2009). Melamine-contaminated milk products induced urinary tract calculi in children. *World J. Pediatr.*, 5(1):31-5.

Zhang Q, Gamboa da Costa G, Von Tungeln LS, Jacob CC, Brown RP, Goering PL. (2012). Urinary biomarker detection of melamine- and cyanuric acid-induced kidney injury in rats. *Toxicol. Sci.*, 129(1):1-8.

Zheng X, Zhao A, Xie G, Chi Y, Zhao L, Li H, Wang C, Bao Y, Jia W, Luther M, Su M, Nicholson JK, Jia W. (2013). Melamine-induced renal toxicity is mediated by the gut microbiota. *Sci. Transl. Med.*, 5(172):172ra22.

In: Fetal Development
Editor: Josiah Wilburn

ISBN: 978-1-63117-069-0

Chapter 5

IMMUNOLOCALIZATION OF SYNTAXIN2 (EPIMORPHIN) IN SINUSOIDAL ENDOTHELIAL CELLS DURING MOUSE LIVER DEVELOPMENT

***Yoshinori Sugiyama*[1], *Tomoaki Tomiya*[2], *Yusuke Akai*[1], *Shunji Hattori*[3], *Toru Koike*[1] and *Nobuyoshi Shiojiri*[1]**

[1]Department of Biology, Faculty of Science, Shizuoka University, Suruga-ku, Shizuoka City, Shizuoka, Japan

[2]Department of Gastroenterology, Faculty of Medicine, University of Tokyo, Bunkyo-ku, Tokyo, Japan

[3]Nippi Research Institute of Biomatrix, Toride City, Ibaraki, Japan

ABSTRACT

Syntaxin2 (epimorphin) expression was immunohistochemically examined during mouse liver development, including the adult stage, with special attention given to hepatic cell types responsible for its production. In the adult liver, nonparenchymal cells in midzonal sinusoidal regions of the lobule had strong positive signals for syntaxin2. Double immunofluorescent analyses using cell type-specific markers demonstrated that sinusoidal endothelial cells expressed syntaxin2 as cytoplasmic granules. Deposition of extracellular matrices such as types I, III and IV collagen, including those around portal and central veins, and in perisinusoidal regions, did not coimmunolocalize with the positive signal of syntaxin2.

In fetal and postnatal livers, the immunolocalization of syntaxin2 was basically similar to that in the adult liver, but its signal in the fetal liver was weak. The expression of syntaxin2 in sinusoidal endothelial cells significantly increased with postnatal liver development. Connective tissues around portal and central veins were mostly negative for syntaxin2 throughout development.

These results suggest that syntaxin2 may be involved in mature functions of sinusoidal endothelial cells, and that it may be one of their good markers in the liver. A monoclonal MC-1 antibody, which was previously shown to react with syntaxin2, stained extracellular fibers of type III collagen around portal and central veins and in the sinusoidal regions of the developing liver and adult liver. Thus, careful consideration is required when the MC-1 antibody is used for immunehistochemistry and loss-of-function experiments with the addition of the antibody. When syntaxin2 was coated on the surface of the dish in the culture of purified fetal hepatoblasts, which are hepatic progenitor cells in the fetal liver, it significantly increased their survival rate and stimulated morphogenesis of spheroid structures. This result suggests that syntaxin2 can act on hepatoblasts for their survival and morphogenesis via a paracrine loop from nonparenchymal cells.

Keywords: Syntaxin2, Epimorphin, Type III collagen, Sinusoid, Liver Development

INTRODUCTION

Epimorphin (also known as syntaxin2) is a unique mesenchymal protein that has morphogenetic effects in multiple epithelial tissues, including those of the mammary gland, lung, pancreas, intestine, and liver, yet its precise mechanisms and in vivo functions remain unknown (Hirai et al., 1992, 1998; Koshida and Hirai, 1997; Lehnert et al., 2001; Oka and Hirai, 1996; Radisky et al., 2003; Simian et al., 2001). Syntaxin2 is a member of the syntaxin family of membrane-bound, intracellular vesicle-docking proteins (Parpura and Mohideen, 2008; Radisky et al., 2003). These proteins are known as target membrane SNAREs (t-SNAREs). Monomeric syntaxin2 (32k) has been detected intracellularly as a component of the SNARE machinery that targets vesicles to the plasma membrane. Although syntaxin2 lacks a signal peptide that directs the protein to extracellular regions, it may translocate across the plasma membrane and be secreted through a non-classical mechanism similar to that described for secretion of the leaderless protein FGF1 (Hirai et al.,, 2007). Syntaxin2 also extracellularly forms an oligomeric form (150k) (Hirai et al., 1992; Hirai, 1994). Recent studies have shown that secreted syntaxin2 binds to αV-integrin-containing receptors on target epithelial cells, leading to activation of specific downstream signaling pathways for epithelial morphogenesis (Hirai et al., 2007).

In the rodent liver, syntaxin2 could be produced by hepatic stellate cells, which control the configuration and gene expression of mature hepatocytes, and has been presumed to localize around hepatic stellate cells (Hirose et al.,, 1996; Yoshino et al., 2006). Syntaxin2 also plays an essential role in the formation of hepatocyte spheroids that maintain differentiated functions in primary culture (Hirose et al., 1996; Watanabe et al., 1998). During liver regeneration after 70% partial hepatectomy or acute liver injury, syntaxin2 expression dramatically changes, suggesting that it may be closely involved in the maintenance of hepatocyte functions or tissue repair (Segawa et al., 2005; Miura et al., 2007; Yoshino et al., 2006). However, it still remains to be accurately demonstrated not only what kind of mechanism is involved in regulation of the histogenesis of hepatocytes by syntaxin2, but also which cells express the protein in the adult liver. It is unknown how the protein is expressed and what kind of role it plays during liver development.

In the present study, the immunolocalization of syntaxin2 was analyzed in adult and developing mouse livers by using an anti-syntaxin2 antibody and monoclonal MC-1 antibody reacting with the protein and canceling its working action (Hirai et al., 1992). Although syntaxin2 was expressed in fetal and postnatal nonparenchymal cells, the MC-1 antigenicity coimmunolocalized with extracellular type III collagen fibers in developing and adult livers. Double immunofluorescent analyses using cell type-specific markers demonstrated that sinusoidal endothelial cells expressed syntaxin2 as cytoplasmic granules in postnatal liver development, which may be involved in their mature functions. Syntaxin2 also significantly increased the survival rate of fetal hepatoblasts and stimulated their morphogenesis of spheroid structures in vitro.

Materials and Methods

Animals

C3H/HeSlc mice (SLC, Hamamatsu, Japan) were used. Animals were mated during the night, and noon of the day the vaginal plug was found was considered 0.5 days of gestation (E0.5). Fetuses at 14.5 and 17.5 days of gestation, newborns (0 day old; P0), and 1-, 2-, 10-week-old (adult) animals were used for immunohistochemistry. At least three animals for each stage, and five sections for each animal were examined in immunohistochemistry. All animal experiments were carried out in compliance with the "Guide for Care and Use of Laboratory Animals" of Shizuoka University.

Immunohistochemistry

Tissues for immunohistochemistry were frozen in liquid nitrogen. Frozen sections were cut at 8 μm thickness and fixed in cold acetone (-20°C) for 10 min. Hydrated sections were incubated with a rabbit anti-rat syntaxin2 antibody (Alomone Labs, Jerusalem, Israel) (1/200 dilution in phosphate-buffered saline [PBS] containing 1% bovine serum albumin [BSA]) and rat monoclonal antibodies against epimorphin (MC-1)(1/200 dilution) for 1 hr at room temperature. After thorough washing with PBS, sections were incubated with a Cy3-labeled donkey anti-rabbit or rat IgG antibody (Jackson ImmunoResearch Lab., West Grove, PA)(1/500 dilution) for 1 hr at room temperature, washed again, and mounted in buffered glycerol containing *p*-phenylenediamine (Johnson and de C Nogueira Araujo, 1981). To examine which cells expressed syntaxin2 and which structures the MC-1 antibody stained in developing and adult livers, double immunofluorescent analyses were carried out for several marker proteins and extracellular matrix components, including E-cadherin (hepatoblasts, hepatocytes and biliary epithelial cells), desmin (stellate cells), vimentin (stellate cells and connective tissue cells), PECAM-1 (endothelial cells), Lyve-1 (endothelial cells), laminin and collagen types I, III and IV (Shiojiri and Sugiyama, 2004), using the primary antibodies listed in Table 1. The following species-specific secondary antibodies were also used: a Cy3 or fluorescein-labeled donkey anti-rabbit, rat or goat IgG antibody (Jackson ImmunoResearch Lab.)(1/500 dilution for Cy3-labeled antibodies and 1/50 dilution for fluorescein-labeled antibodies).

Table 1. Primary antibodies used in immunohistochemistry

Antibody	Source	Dilution
Goat anti-human desmin antibody (Y-20)	Santa Cruz Biotechnology, Inc., Santa Cruz, CA	1:200
Goat anti-rat type III collagen antiserum	(Nakanishi et al., 1988)	1:100
Goat anti-vimentin antiserum	ICN Biochemicals, Aurora, OH	1:100
Rabbit anti-chicken desmin antiserum	Progen Biotechnik Gmbh, Heidelberg, Germany	1:100
Rabbit anti-mouse carbamoylphosphate synthase I (CPSI) antibody	(Nitou et al., 2002)	1:500
Rabbit anti-mouse laminin antiserum	E-Y Lab., San Mateo, CA	1:100
Rabbit anti-mouse type IV collagen antiserum	Chemicon International, Temecula, CA	1:100
Rabbit anti-rat syntaxin2 antiserum	Alomone Labs, Jerusalem, Israel	1:200
Rabbit anti-rat type I collagen antiserum	Chemicon International, Temecula, CA	1:100
Rabbit anti-rat type III collagen antiserum	Chemicon International, Temecula, CA	1:100
Rat anti-mouse E-cadherin antibody (ECCD-2)	Takara Biomedical, Otsu, Japan	1:100
Rat anti-mouse epimorphin antibody (MC-1 monoclonal)	(Hirai et al., 1992)	1:200
Rat anti-mouse Lyve-1 antibody (Xb-13)	Santa Cruz Biotechnology, Inc., Santa Cruz, CA	1:200
Rat anti-mouse PECAM-1 antibody	eBioscience, San Diego, CA	1:100

Control incubations were carried out in PBS containing 1% BSA in place of the primary antibodies. Nuclei were stained with DAPI in some cases.

Immunoblotting

Pieces of adult mouse livers were homogenized in a lysis buffer containing 10mM Tris-HCl (pH 7.8), 1% Nonidet P-40, 150mM NaCl, 0.1% sodium dodecyl sulfate (SDS), 0.5% sodium deoxycholate and protease inhibitors. After lysates were centrifuged at 11,000g for 10 min, the supernatant was collected and the concentration of protein was determined using a BCA protein assay reagent kit (Pierce Chemical Company, Rockford, IL). Lysates (20 μg), and human and bovine type III collagens (20 μg) reduced by the method of Laemmli [1970] were electrophoresed on SDS-7% polyacrylamide gel. Proteins in the gel were transferred to PVDF membranes (Immobilon-P; Millipore Corp., Billeria, MA). The membranes were blocked with 5% skim milk in Tris-HCl (pH 7.4)-buffered saline containing 0.1% Tween 20 (TBST). After washing with TBST, incubation with the primary antibody (anti-type III collagen [1/1000 dilution] and MC-1 antibody [1/1000 dilution]) was performed overnight at 4°C. Following washing with TBST, the membranes were incubated with a horseradish peroxidase-labeled goat anti-rabbit or rat IgG antibody (Jackson ImmunoResearch Lab.)(1/2000 dilution) for 2 hrs at room temperature. ECL detection was conducted with Amersham Pharmacia Biotech (Buckinghamshire, UK) reagents according to the manufacturer's recommendations.

In Vitro Culture

Briefly, 12.5-day (E12.5) fetal livers were diced and treated with dispase (1000U/mL) (Godo Shusei, Tokyo, Japan) in Dulbecco's modified Eagle's medium (DMEM)(Gibco, Grand Island, NY) containing 10% fetal bovine serum (FBS) for 30 min at 37°C (Nitou et al., 2002; Sugiyama et al., 2007). The liver specimens were subsequently dispersed into single cells by mild pipetting, and filtrated through a nylon mesh filter (pore size 132 μm) (Nihon Rikagaku Kikai, Tokyo, Japan). The filtrate was centrifuged at 50xg for 10 min. The cellular pellet was washed twice with DM-160 (Kyokuto Seiyaku, Tokyo, Japan) containing 10% FBS and 0.01% deoxyribonuclease I (Worthington Biochem. Corp., Freehold, NJ). The resulting cellular pellet was resuspended in DM-160 supplemented with 10% FBS, dexamethasone (10^{-7}M) and antibiotics, and prepared at a cell density of 10^6 cells/mL. The fetal liver cells (10^6 cells/mL, 70 μL) were cultured on a glass area (a diameter of 6 mm) surrounded by a Teflon-coated area on glass slides (AR Brown, Tokyo, Japan) at 37°C in a water-saturated atmosphere containing 5% CO_2. E12.5 hepatoblasts were purified by using anti-E-cadherin antibody-coated magnetic beads (Nitou et al., 2002), and cultured on dishes coated with several extracellular matrix components, including bovine type I collagen (20 μg/cm^2), mouse type IV collagen (BD Biosciences, Bedford, MA)(10 μg/cm^2), mouse fibronectin (Chemicon)(2 μg/cm^2), mouse laminin (BD Biosciences) (10 μg/cm^2) or syntaxin2 (recombinant epimorphin [2-5 μg/cm^2])(Hirai et al., 1998). Syntaxin2 (soluble recombinant epimorphin [Hirai et al., 1998]) was added to the culture medium in some cultures of purified hepatoblasts (100 μg/mL).

The conditioned medium prepared from the culture of E12.5 liver cells (Nitou et al., 2002) or a rat hepatic stellate cell line (CFSC-8B)(Greenwel et al., 1993) was also added to the culture of purified hepatoblasts at a concentration of 20-30%. For immunohistochemistry, the cultured cells were fixed in cold acetone for 10 min.

RESULTS

Expression of Syntaxin2 in the Adult Liver

The syntaxin2 antibody reacted with sinusoidal cells in the adult mouse liver, showing a zonal distribution with almost no expression in periportal or pericentral sinusoidal cells (Figure 1a, b). Sinusoidal cells in the middle zone of the hepatic lobule had a tendency to show stronger syntaxin2 expression. The syntaxin2-positive signals took a granular morphology in the cytoplasm of the sinusoidal cells (Figure 1c, d). Mature hepatocytes, biliary epithelial cells, and cells of portal veins and central veins were not reactive to the anti-syntaxin2 antibody.

In order to demonstrate which cells express syntaxin2 for stellate cells or endothelial cells constituting hepatic sinusoids, double immunofluorescent analyses were carried out. As a result, the immunolocalization of syntaxin2 was often closely located with the positive signals of desmin or vimentin, which were used as a marker of stellate cells, but both positive signals rarely coimmunolocalized (Figure 2a-c). In addition to the sinusoidal regions, desmin-positive signals were detectable in connective tissues cells of portal and central veins whereas syntaxin2 expression was totally absent in these regions (Figure 2b, c). By contrast, the immunolocalizations of PECAM-1 or Lyve-1, which were used as a marker of endothelial cells, well overlapped with the syntaxin2-positive signals in sinusoids (Figure 2d-i), indicating that sinusoidal endothelial cells, but not stellate cells, expressed syntaxin2.

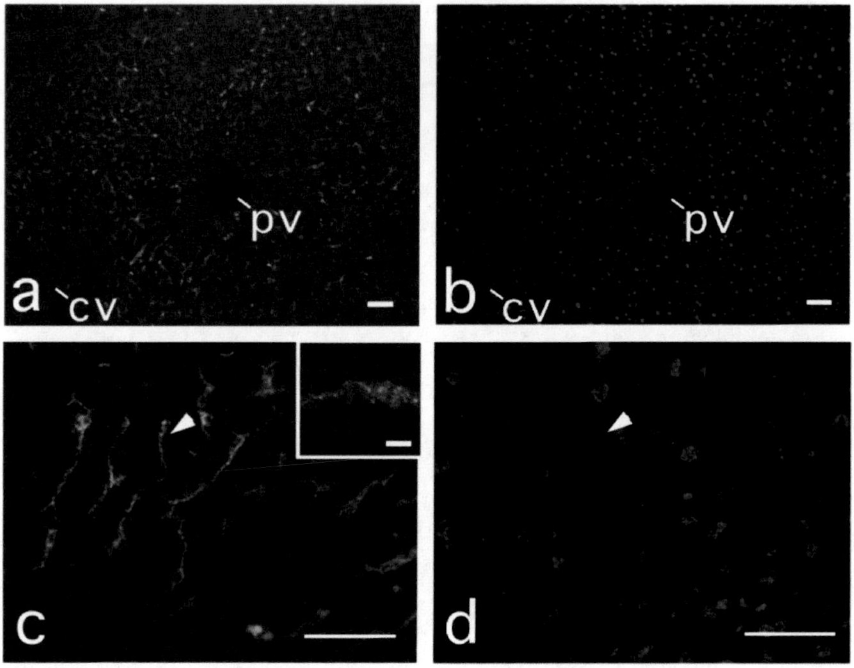

Figure 1. Immunohistochemical analysis of syntaxin2 expression in adult liver. a, c. Syntaxin2 immunofluorescenc. b, d. DAPI staining in a and c, respectively. Syntaxin2 immunolocalizes at sinusoidal cells variably within hepatic lobule (a-d; arrowheads in c and d). Granular immunofluorescence is seen in sinusoidal cells (inset in c). cv, central vein; pv, portal vein. Bars in a-d indicate 50 μm. Bar in a inset of c indicates 6 μm.

Next, the correlation between the distribution of syntaxin2-positive cells and hepatic zonation of E-cadherin expression in mature hepatocytes was examined. E-cadherin and N-cadherin was complementarily expressed in the hepatic lobule (Doi et al., 2007).Double immunofluorescent analyses demonstrated that the distribution of syntaxin2-positive cells had no correlation with periportal E-cadherin expression (Figure 3a-f). Syntaxin2-positive cells were often close to those of extracellular matrix components, including types I, III and IV collagen and laminin, in sinusoidal regions, which were more abundantly deposited in portal connective tissues that were negative for syntaxin2 expression (Figure 4a, b). There was no correlation between syntaxin2 expression and these extracellular matrix deposition.

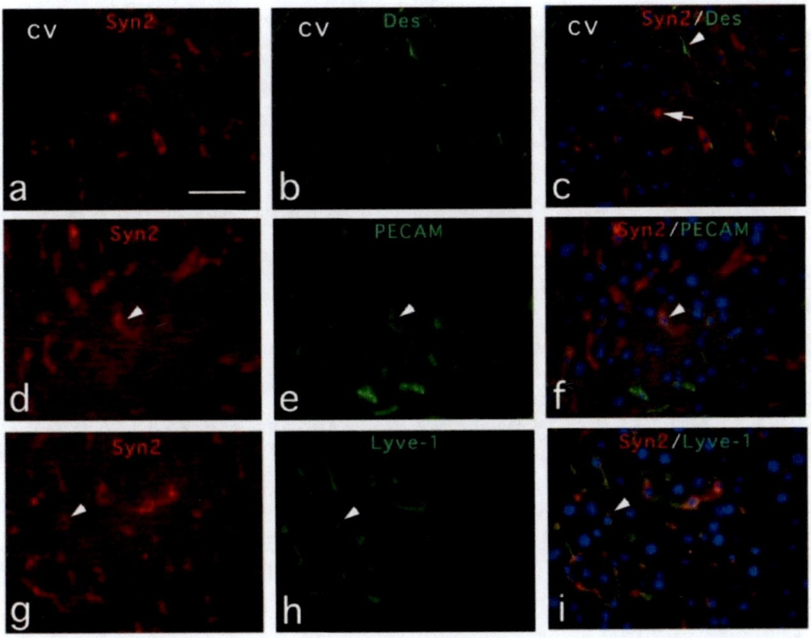

Figure 2. Double immunofluorescent analysis of syntaxin2 (red; a, c, d, f, g, i) and desmin (green; b, c), PECAM-1 (green; e, f) or Lyve-1 expression (green; h, i) in adult livers. c, f, i. Merged photographs of a and b, d and e, and g and h, respectively. DAPI staining (blue) is also merged. Although syntaxin2-positive signals in sinusoidal cells are closely located to desmin signals in stellate cells in most cases, both signals do not merge precisely (a-c). Desmin-positive cells without any syntaxin2-negative signals are seen (arrowhead). Isolated syntaxin2-positive signals are also seen (arrow). Syntaxin2-positive signals in sinusoidal cells (d, g) overlap with those of PECAM-1 (e, f) or Lyve-1 (h, i)(arrowheads). cv, central vein. Bar indicates 50 μm.

Immunolocalization of Syntaxin 2 during Liver Development

Syntaxin2 was not immunohistochemically detectable in E12.5 livers. In the E14.5 liver, nonparenchymal cells between hepatic cords were weakly reactive (Figure 5a-c; Table 2). After birth, the syntaxin2 immunoreactivity in nonparenchymal cells increased, and sinusoidal cells became strongly positive in the P7 and P14 liver as seen in the adult liver (Figure 5d-1). Some positive cells were detectable in portal connective tissues in neonatal livers. Double immunofluorescent analysis of syntaxin2 and Lyve-1 or PECAM-1 demonstrated that sinusoidal endothelial cells expressed syntaxin2 in P7 and P14 livers (Figure 6a-i).

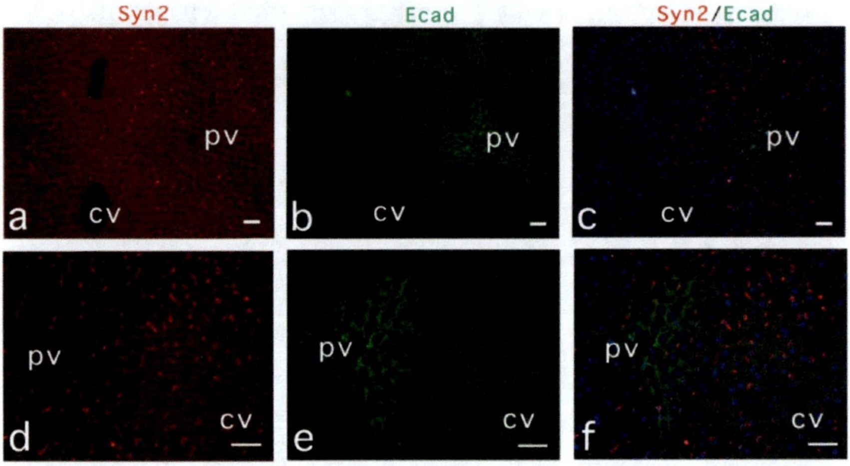

Figure 3. Heterogeneous distribution of syntaxin2-positive sinusoidal cells is not dependent on zonal expression of E-cadherin in hepatic lobules. a, d. Syntaxin2 immunofluorescence. b, e. E-cadherin immunofluorescence. c, f. Merged photographs of a and b, and d and e, respectively. DAPI staining (blue) is also shown. Although syntaxin2 expression has a tendency to be strong in the middle zone of the hepatic lobule, that pattern does not depend on the heterogeneous (portal) expression of E-cadherin. cv, central vein; pv, portal vein. Bars indicate 50 μm.

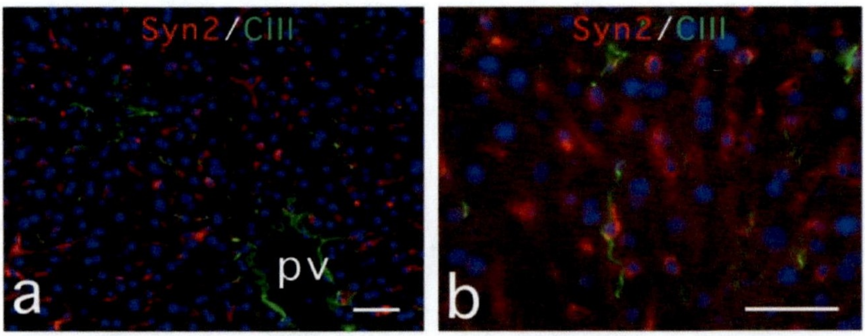

Figure 4. Double immunofluorescent analysis of type III collagen (green) and syntaxin2 (red) in adult liver. a, b. Merged photographs of type III collagen, syntaxin2 and DAPI. Both antigens are detectable in sinusoidal regions but do not merge (a, b). Whereas type III collagen is abundantly detectable in connective tissues of a portal vein, syntaxin2 is not observed. pv, portal vein. Bars indicate 50 μm.

Some Lyve-1-negative or PECAM-1-negative cells in sinusoids expressed syntaxin2 in these livers. Endothelial cells of portal and central veins were negative for syntaxin2 throughout liver development.

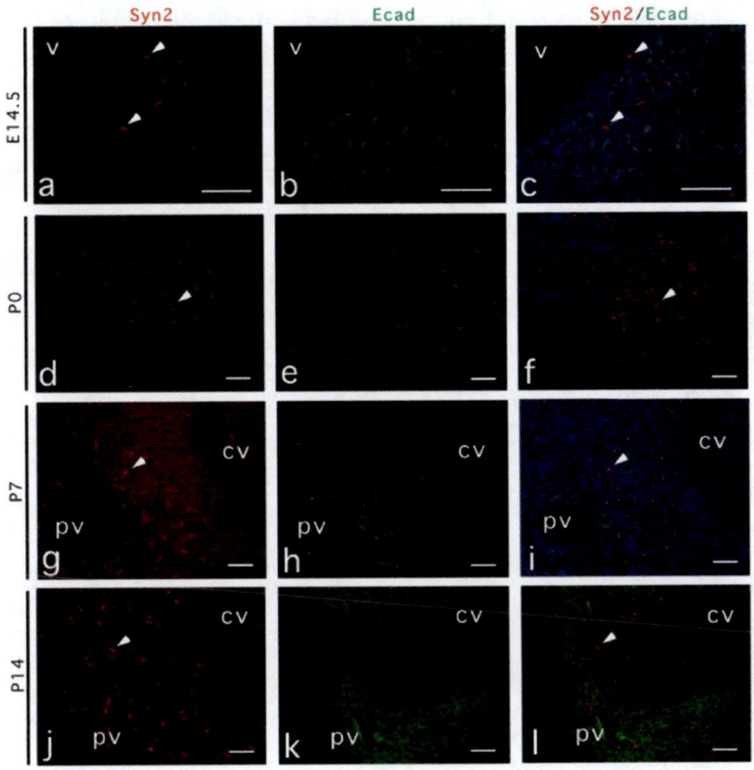

Figure 5. Immunohistochemical analysis of syntaxin2 expression (a, d, g, j) during liver development. a-c. E14.5 liver. d-f. P0 liver. g-i. P7 liver. j-l. P14 liver. b, e, h, k. E-cadherin expression in a, d, g, and j, respectively. c, f, i, l. Merged photographs of a and b, d and e, g and h, and j and k, respectively. DAPI fluorescence (blue) is also shown. In an E14.5 liver, syntaxin2 signals are not abundant (a-c). In a neonatal liver, syntaxin2-positive signals are detectable in sinusoidal areas (d-f). In P7 and P14 livers, heterogeneous expression pattern of syntaxin2 starts to be established (g-l). Arrowheads indicate syntaxin2-positive cells. cv, central vein; pv, portal vein. Bars indicate 50 μm.

Immunolocalization of MC-1 Antigenicity during Liver Development

In the adult liver, positive MC-1 immunoreaction was detectable in sinusoidal regions and connective tissues around portal and central veins (Figure 7a-c). It also appeared to be fibrous and extracellular in single immunehistochemistry for the MC-1 antibody. Desmin and vimentin expression in stellate cells did not coimmunolocalize with signals of the MC-1 antigen in most cases (Figure 7b, c). The MC-1 antigen was often observed in regions where desmin or vimentin-positive cells were absent.

Table 2. Developmental changes of syntaxin2 expression during mouse liver development

Cell type	E14.5	E17.5	P0	P7	P14	Adult
Hepatoblasts/Hepatocytes	-	-	-	-	-	-
Biliary epithelial cells	-	-	-	-	-	-
Stellate cells	*	*	*	-	-	-
Endothelial cells (sinusoid)	-/±	-/±	-/±	-/++	-/++	-/++
Endothelial cells (portal vein)	-	-	-	-	-	-
Endothelial cells (central vein)	-	-	-	-	-	-
Connective tissue (portal vein)	-	-	-/+	-	-	-
[a]Other cells	-/±	-/±	-/±	-	*	*

P0, newborns; P7 and P14, 7-day-old and 14-day-old mice, respectively. [a]Other cells include hemopoietic cells. *, not examined. ++, strong immunofluorescence; +, moderate immunofluorescence; ±, weak immunofluorescence; -, no immunofluorescence; -/+, moderately fluorescent cells and nonfluorescent cells.

Immunoreactivity to the MC-1 antibody was also observed in connective tissues around portal veins and central veins, and in sinusoidal regions throughout liver development (Figure 7d-f). Although, on day 12.5, the immunoreactivity was not abundant, the positive signals took the form of fibrous deposition but they did not always agree with the distribution of stellate cells that expressed desmin or vimentin (Figure 7d). Although MC-1-positive fibers were often deposited near stellate cells, they were also seen in the regions where desmin-positive stellate cells were absent. PECAM-1-positive sinusoidal endothelial cells were supported by MC-1-positive fibrous materials. With liver development, the MC-1 immunoreactivity increased in perisinusoidal regions and around portal and central veins. Double immunofluorescent analyses of the MC-1 antibody and antibodies against extracellular matrix components demonstrated that the distribution of type IV collagen was close to that of MC-1 antigenicity, but their immunoreactivities did not perfectly merge in developing and adult livers (Figure 7h, k).

The immunolocalization of type I collagen partly coimmunolocalized with that of MC-1 reactivity, especially in the sinusoidal regions, but that around large vessels did not overlap with the MC-1 reactivity (Figure 7g, j). However, type III collagen perfectly coimmunolocalized with the MC-1 antigenicity throughout liver development, including the adult stage (Figure 7i, l).

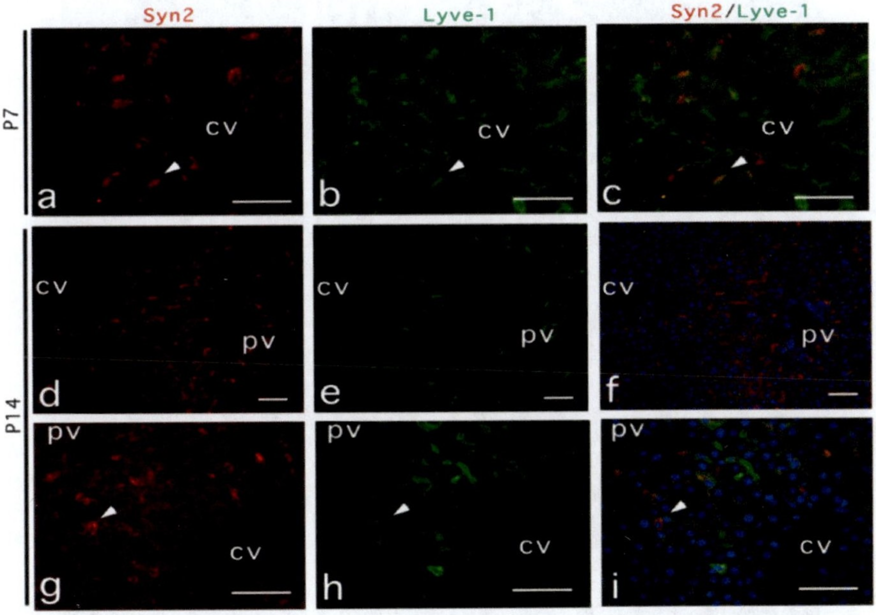

Figure 6. Sinusoidal endothelial cells express syntaxin2 during postnatal liver development. a-c. P7 liver. d-i. P14 livers. a, d, g. Syntaxin2 immunofluorescence. b, e, h. Lyve-1 expression in a, d, and g, respectively. c, f, i. Merged photographs of a and b, d and e, and g and h, respectively. DAPI fluorescence (blue) is also shown. Arrowheads indicate syntaxin2-positive and Lyve-1-positive cells (a-c, g-i). Lyve-1-positive cells overlap with syntaxin2-positive cells (a-i). cv, central vein; pv, portal vein. Bars indicate 50 μm.

Specificities of MC-1 Antibody

Immunoblotting analysis using MC-1 antibody demonstrated that that antibody detected a 150k protein band in adult liver lysates (Figure 8a). The antibody was also clearly reactive with 140k bands of human and bovine type III collagens (Figure 8a). It weakly reacted with several bands, including those with a molecular weight of 30k. The anti-type III collagen antibody used for immunohistochemistry in the present study was specifically reactive with bovine and human type III collagens (Figure 8b). It also reacted strongly with a 150k protein band and weakly with several protein bands in adult liver extracts like the MC-1 antibody.

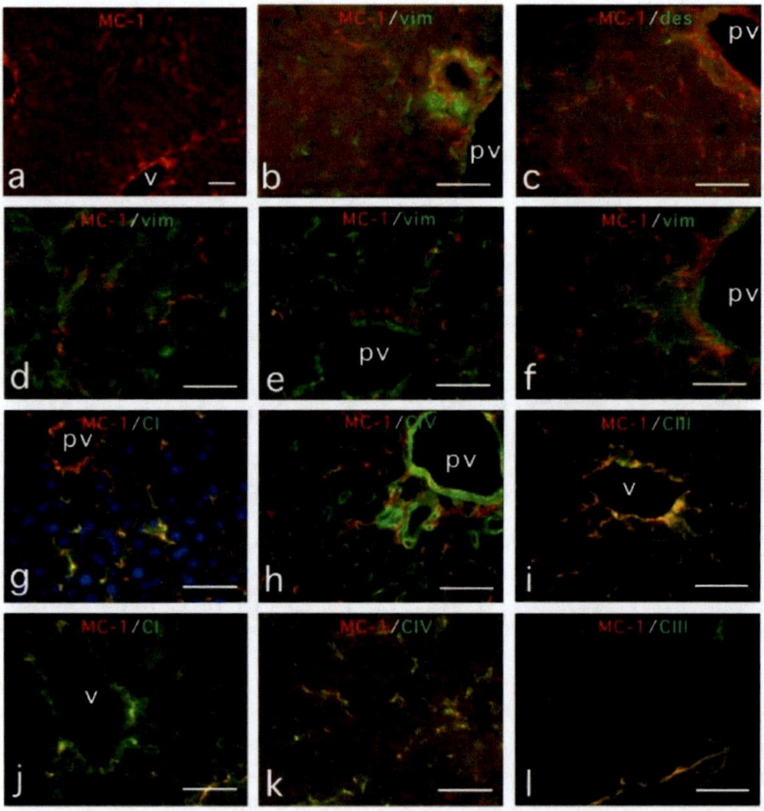

Figure 7. Immunolocalization of MC-1 antigenicity (red) during liver development. a-c, g-i. Adult liver. d. E12.5 liver. e. E17.5 liver. f. P0 liver. j-l. E14.5 liver. a-c. In adult liver, MC-1 antigenicity is immunolocalized to nonparenchymal regions as fibers, and is located very close to vimentin- (green, b) or desmin- (green, c) positive stellate cells. d-f. MC-1 antigenicity is present around large blood vessels or in sinusoidal regions in E12.5, E17.5 and P0 livers. Green, vimentin immunofluorescence. g-l. Double immunofluorescent analyses of MC-1 and type I collagen (green)(g, j), type IV collagen (green) (h, k) or type III collagen (green) (i, l) in adult liver (g-i) and E14.5 (j-l) liver. Although the MC-1 immunolocalization resembles those of type I and type IV collagen, they do not perfectly overlap (g, h, j, k). By contrast, the MC-1 immunolocalization perfectly overlaps with that of type III collagen (i, l). pv, portal vein; v, vessel. Bars indicate 50 μm.

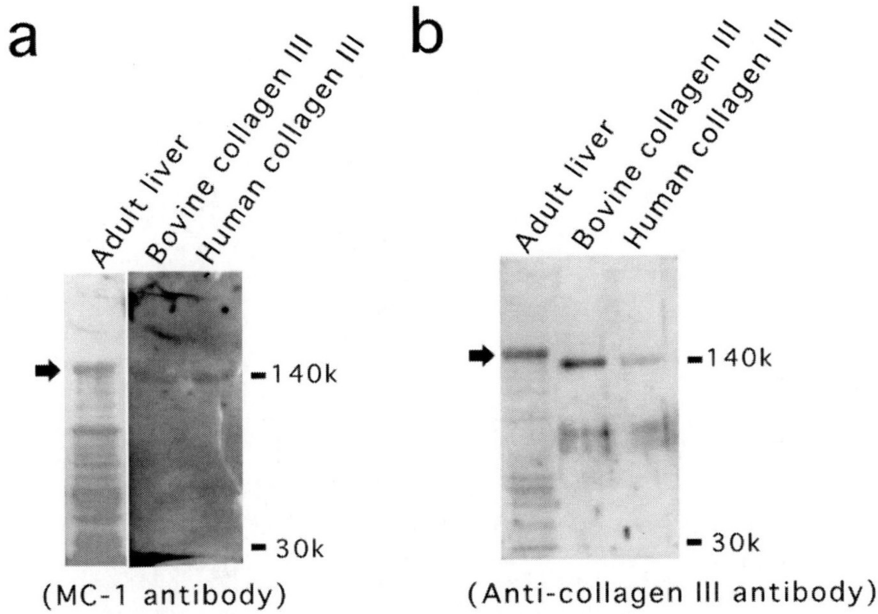

Figure 8. Immunoblotting analysis for specificity of MC-1 antibody. a. MC-1 antibody reacts mainly with a 150k band in adult liver cell lysate (arrow), and also with bands of 140k bovine and human type III collagen. MC-1 antibody is also weakly reactive with several bands, including those with a molecular weight of approximately 30k in the cell lysate. b. Anti-rat type III collagen antibody reacts mainly with 140k bands of bovine and human type III collagens, and with a 150k band of type III collagen in adult liver cell lysate (arrow).

Effects of Syntaxin2 and Extracellular Matrix Components on Survival and Morphogenesis of Hepatoblasts

Primary hepatocytes from adult rat livers have been shown to be stimulated to construct spheroidal structures having high hepatic functions in vitro (Hirose et al., 1996; Watanabe et al., 1998). We examined whether syntaxin2 promotes the histogenesis of hepatoblasts, which are hepatic progenitor cells in the fetal liver, or not. Hepatoblasts were isolated from E12.5 liver cell suspensions by anti-E-cadherin antibody-coated magnetic beads and cultured on the dishes coated with several extracelluar matrix components or syntaxin2 (Figures 9, 10).

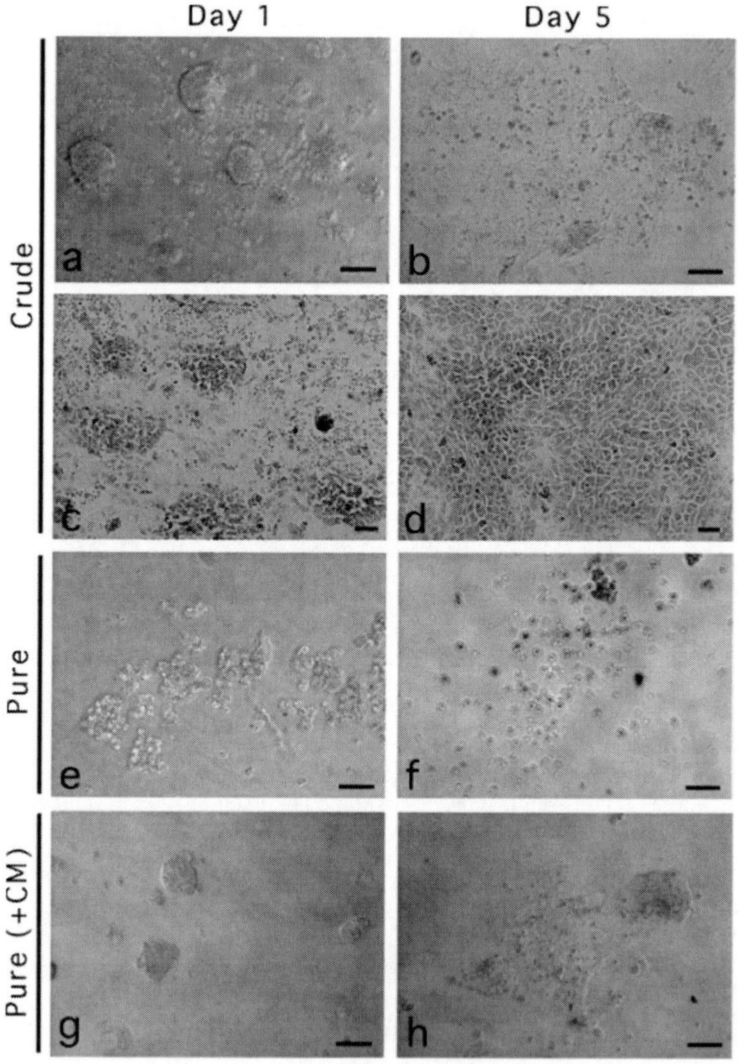

Figure 9. Fetal hepatoblasts form round aggregates in the presence of nonparenchymal cells (crude culture) or conditioned medium (CM). E12.5 liver cells were cultured in vitro for 1 (a, c, e, g) or 5 days (b, d, f, h). a, b, e-h. Phase-contrast micrograph. c, d. H-E staining. Hepatoblasts form spherical aggregates on day 1 (a, c), and spread on the glass slide on day 5 (b, d) in the presence of nonparenchymal cells. Purified hepatoblasts aggregate loosely on day 1 (e), and are dead on day 5 (f). The presence of the conditioned medium supported purified hepatoblasts to form round aggregates on day 1 (g), and to survive and spread on the glass slide on day 5 (h). Bars indicate 50 μm.

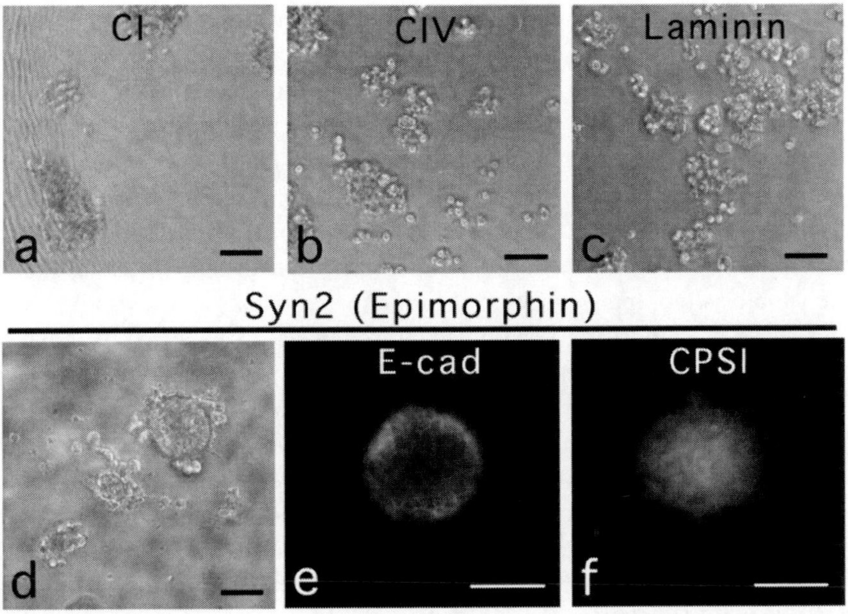

Figure 10. Syntaxin2 supports hepatoblast survival and morphogenesis of spherical aggregates in vitro. Purified hepatoblasts were cultured for 1 day on glass slides coated with type I collagen (a), type IV collagen (b), laminin (c) and syntaxin2 (d). a-d. Phase-contrast micrograph. e, f. E-cadherin and carbamoylphosphate synthase I immunohistochemistry, respectively. Although coating of type I collagen (a) stimulated the adhesion of hepatoblasts to the glass slide, it did not support their formation of round aggregates and survival. Coating of type IV collagen (b) and laminin (c) has no effect on hepatoblast adhesion and formation of round aggregates by purified hepatoblasts in the absence of nonparenchymal cells or conditioned medium. Syntaxin2 induces hepatoblasts to form round aggregates (d). Hepatoblasts forming round aggregates on syntaxin2-coated glass slides express E-cadherin (e) and carbamoylphosphate synthase I (f). Bars indicate 50 μm.

When purified hepatoblasts were again recombined and cultured with nonparenchymal cells on the glass slide, they formed spherical aggregates, which were supported by hepatic stellate cells and firmly attached to the glass slide on day 1 (Figure 9a, c). Thereafter, they grew on the glass slide and expressed hepatic functions (data not shown) concomitantly with remarkable growth of nonparenchymal cells (especially desmin-positive stellate cells)(Figure 9b, d). In the absence of nonparenchymal cells, hepatoblasts of the aggregates died without firm adhesion to the glass slide (Figure 9e, f). Their cell-cell adhesion was loose. The conditioned medium from cultures of E12.5 liver cells and the stellate cell line significantly supported the survival, growth and maturation of purified hepatoblasts in vitro as well as in their coculture with nonparenchymal cells (Figure 9g, h). The coating of the culture glass slide with syntaxin2 (recombinant epimorphin) or the addition of syntaxin2 to the culture medium significantly supported the survival of hepatoblasts, and stimulated the formation of spheroids by hepatoblasts expressing E-cadherin and carbamoylphosphate synthase I on day 1 (Figure 10d-f). Although almost all experiments using syntaxin2 had round spheroid formation (ten cultures showing spheroid formation in ten experiments), not all hepatoblasts took part in spheroid formation. In addition, it did not support longer survival of purified hepatoblasts through day 5 in vitro. By contrast, coating of extracellular matrix components on the glass slide did not support the survival of hepatoblasts in the absence of nonparenchymal cells or the conditioned medium (no culture showing spheroid formation in twenty experiments using various extracellular matrix components)(Figure 10a-c), though almost all hepatoblasts firmly adhered to the coated glass slide, especially that coated with type I collagen and fibronectin. Even in these cases, hepatoblasts did not form ball-like spheroids, and had a shape of aggregates like a bunch of grapes via their loose adhesion.

DISCUSSION

The present study demonstrated that syntaxin2 (epimorphin) was expressed in sinusoids in adult and postnatal developing mouse livers, and that the endothelial cells, but not stellate cells, were responsible for their production. These data are not consistent with those by Watanabe et al., [1998] showing that syntaxin2 (MC-1 antigen) localizes at the surface of hepatic stellate cells residing in perisinusoidal spaces with a MC-1 monoclonal antibody that was reported to specifically react with syntaxin2 (epimorphin), especially an oligomeric form of syntaxin2 with an approximate molecular weight of 150k (Hirai et al., 1992). The present study also showed that both syntaxin2 and MC-1 antigen did not coimmunolocalize in sinusoids of adult and developing livers. Double immunofluorescent analyses using the MC-1 antibody and antibodies against extracellular matrix proteins demonstrated that type III collagen coimmunolocalized with the MC-1 antigen in sinusoidal areas and connective tissues of portal and central veins. Furthermore, the MC-1 antibody that we used in our immunohistochemistry reacted with bovine and human type III collagens with a molecular weight of 140k in immunoblotting analysis. These data clearly indicated that the MC-1 antibody detected type III collagen in tissue sections of mouse organs. Our anti-syntaxin2 antibody did not react with type III collagen in tissue sections and immunoblotting (data, not shown). The molecular size of the band that was detectable by the MC-1 antibody in immunoblotting analysis of cell lysates of adult livers, including anti-rat type III collagen antibody, was 150k, which corresponds to that of syntaxin2 (epimorphin) detected in several tissues, including embryonic skin and lung (Hirai et al., 1992), but may be larger than the molecular weight of mouse type III collagen (140k). This difference may be explained by our inadequate extraction protocol for type III collagen. Normally, type III collagen can be extracted by acid treatment or protease pretreatment (Bornstein and Traub, 1979; Sato et al., 2000), but not by detergent treatment such as that with SDS carried out in the present study. The molecules of the band with a molecular weight of 150k may be type III collagen-like molecules, including the pro-form of type III collagen. In any event, the MC-1 antibody may strongly react with type III collagen in immunohistochemistry and immunoblotting. Therefore, considering the immunolocalization of syntaxin2 (epimorphin) and loss-of-function experiments using the MC-1 antibody, special caution should be paid. It may be still possible that the MC-1 antibody reacts with epimorphin (syntaxin2) in addition to type III collagen, because it reacted with low molecular weight bands in our immunoblotting data of adult liver cell lysates. However, these bands might have been degraded products of type III collagen molecules.

Syntaxin2 was strongly expressed as cytoplasmic granules in sinusoidal endothelial cells of middle zones of the hepatic lobule, implying that it may function as a component of the SNARE machinery that targets vesicles to the plasma membrane. Furthermore, sinusoidal syntaxin2 expression significantly increased with postnatal liver development, which suggests that this may be related to an acquisition of mature function by sinusoidal endothelial cells. Heterogeneous expression of syntaxin2 and also Lyve-1 in the hepatic lobule indicates the heterogeneous functional states of sinusoidal endothelial cells, which may have some influences on the hepatic zonation of heterogeneous gene expression of hepatocytes (Gebhardt and Mecke, 1983; Stanulović et al., 2007). The staining intensities of syntaxin2 and Lyve-1 were not always consistent in endothelial cell population, suggesting that each endothelial cell is in different functional states. It is also noteworthy that syntaxin2 expression is detectable only in endothelial cells of sinusoids, but not in those of portal veins and central veins. This result indicates that syntaxin2 expression may be one of good markers characterizing sinusoidal endothelial cells in addition to Lyve-1 expression in the adult liver.

The present study demonstrated that the addition of syntaxin2 to the culture of purified hepatoblasts significantly stimulated their viability and morphogenesis as a spheroid, though it was not sufficient for full survival of hepatoblasts as seen in cultures with the addition of the conditioned medium or the presence of nonparenchymal cells. Primary hepatocytes from adult rat livers were stimulated to construct spheroidal structures having high hepatic functions when it was added to the culture medium (Hirose et al., 1996; Watanabe et al., 1998). Although it is unknown how exogenous syntaxin2 works on hepatoblasts or hepatocytes, mechanisms such as syntaxin-αV-integrin-FAK signaling, which leads to cell survival pathways, might be involved in this phenomenon (Hirai et al., 2007). Because sinusoidal endothelial cells, but not stellate cells, adjoining hepatoblasts or hepatocytes, expressed syntaxin2 during liver development, they may provide syntaxin2 to hepatoblasts and hepatocytes for their survival and morphogenesis in vivo. As their syntaxin2 expression was prominent in postnatal livers, including the adult liver, syntaxin2 may act on the organization of hepatic architecture in postnatal stages such as liver lobule formation and sinusoid maturation. Syntaxin2 may also be expressed in a small amount in the young fetal liver or masked in our tissue sections of E12.5 and E14.5 livers, and work on survival and morphogenesis of hepatoblasts.

It is also of note that the extracellular matrix components did not work as a primary survival factor for purified hepatoblasts as compared with the action of syntaxin2. Although purified hepatoblasts could firmly adhere to the type I collagen- or fibronectin-coated dishes, the coating did not enhance the viability of the hepatoblasts. By contrast, the conditioned media prepared from conventional cultures of E12.5 liver cells or the hepatic stellate cell line were highly stimulatory for the hepatoblast survival, growth and gene expression. It would be intriguing to identify what molecules such stimulatory factors are. As the medium from the hepatic stellate cell line can be collected in a large amount (Greenwel et al., 1993), it will be helpful for purification of effective factors.

CONCLUSION

Sinusoidal endothelial cells express syntaxin2 as cytoplasmic granules in postnatal liver development, which may be involved in their mature functions. Syntaxin2 is also weakly expressed in nonparenchymal cells at fetal stages, significantly increases the survival rate of fetal hepatoblasts and stimulates their morphogenesis of spheroid structures in vitro. A monoclonal MC-1 antibody, which was previously shown to react with syntaxin2, stains extracellular fibers of type III collagen in the developing liver and adult liver. Careful consideration is required when this antibody is used for immunohistochemistry and loss-of-function experiments.

ACKNOWLEDGMENT

We thank Professor Emeritus Takeo Mizuno of the University of Tokyo and Prof. Nelson Fausto of the University of Washington for their interest in our study and encouragement, and Mr. Kim Barrymore for his help in preparing our manuscript. We also thank Drs. Yohei Hirai and Yasuo Nakanishi for their kind gift of the MC-1 antibody and anti-type III collagen antiserum, respectively. This work was performed in part through Special Coordination Funds for Promoting Science and Technology from the Ministry of Education, Culture, Sports, Science and Technology, the Japanese Government, a Grant for Child Health and Development (17C-4) from the Ministry of Health, Labor and Welfare, the Japanese Government, a Grant-in-Aid from the Ministry of Education, Culture, Sports, Science and Technology, Japan (number 19570203), and a grant from the Sumitomo Foundation (number 060110).

REFERENCES

Bornstein P. and Traub W. (1979) The chemistry and biology of collagen. In: The Proteins, Vol. IV, edited by Naurath H. and Hill R. L., Academic Press, New York, pp411-632.

Doi Y., Tamura S., Nammo T., Fukui K., Kiso S. and Nagafuchi A. (2007) Development of complementary expression patterns of E- and N-cadherin in the mouse liver. *Hepatol. Res.*, 37, 230-237.

Gebhardt R. and Mecke D. (1983) Heterogeneous distribution of glutamine synthetase among rat liver parenchymal cells in situ and in primary culture. *EMBO J.,* 2, 567-570.

Greenwel P., Rubin J., Schwartz M., Hertzberg E. L. and Rojkind M. (1993) Liver fat-storing cell clones obtained from a CCl4-cirrhotic rat are heterogeneous with regard to proliferation, expression of extracellular matrix components, interleukin-6, and connexin 43. *Lab. Invest.*, 69, 210-216.

Hirai Y. (1994) Sodium-dodecyl-sulfate-resistant complex formation of epimorphin monomers and interaction of the 150-kDa complex with the cell surface. *Eur. J. Biochem.*, 225, 1133-1139.

Hirai Y., Takebe K., Takashina M., Kobayashi S. and Takeichi M. (1992) Epimorphin: a mesenchymal protein essential for epithelial morphogenesis. *Cell*, 69, 471-481.

Hirai Y., Lochter A., Galosy S., Koshida S., Niwa S. and Bissell M. J. (1998) Epimorphin functions as a key morphoregulator for mammary epithelial cells. *J. Cell Biol.,* 140, 159-169.

Hirai Y., Nelson C. M., Yamazaki K., Takebe K., Przybylo J., Madden B. and Radisky D. C. (2007) Non-classical export of epimorphin and its adhesion to αv-integrin in regulation of epithelial morphogenesis. *J. Cell Sci.,* 120, 2032-2043.

Hirose M., Watanabe S., Oide H., Kitamura T., Miyazaki A. and Sato N. (1996) A new function of Ito cells in liver morphogenesis: evidence using a novel morphogenic protein, epimorphin, in vitro. *Biochem. Biophys. Res. Commun.*, 225, 155-160.

Johnson G. D. and de C Nogueira Araujo G. M. (1981) A simple method of reducing the fading of immunofluorescence during microscopy. *J. Immunol. Methods,* 43, 349-350.

Koshida S. and Hirai Y. (1997) Identification of cellular recognition sequence of epimorphin and critical role of cell/epimorphin interaction in lung branching morphogenesis. *Biochem. Biophys. Res. Commun.*, 234, 522-525.

Laemmli U. K. (1970) Cleavage of structural proteins during the assembly of the head of bacteriophage T4. *Nature,* 227, 680-685.

Lehnert L., Lerch M. M., Hirai Y., Kruse M. L., Schmiegel W. and Kalthoff H. (2001) Autocrine stimulation of human pancreatic duct-like development by soluble isoforms of epimorphin in vitro. *J. Cell Biol.*, 152, 911-922.

Miura K., Yoshino R., Hirai Y., Goto T., Ohshima S., Mikami K., Yoneyama K., Watanabe D., Sato M., Senoo H., Kodama Y., Osawa Y., Brenner D. A. and Watanabe S. (2007) Epimorphin, a morphogenic protein, induces proteases in rodent hepatocytes through NF-kappaB. *J. Hepatol.*, 47, 834-843.

Nakanishi Y., Nogawa H., Hashimoto Y., Kishi J. and Hayakawa T. (1988) Accumulation of collagen III at the cleft points of developing mouse submandibular epithelium. *Development*, 104, 51-59.

Nitou M., Sugiyama Y., Ishikawa K. and Shiojiri N. (2002) Isolation of hepatoblasts from fetal mouse liver with magnetic beads coated with anti-E-cadherin antibodies. *Exp. Cell Res.*, 279, 330-343.

Oka Y. and Hirai Y. (1996) Inductive influences of epimorphin on endothelial cells in vitro. *Exp. Cell Res.*, 222, 189-198.

Parpura V. and Mohideen U. (2008) Molecular form follows function: (un)snaring the SNAREs. *Trends Neurosci.*, 31, 435-443.

Radisky D. C., Hirai Y. and Bissell M. J. (2003) Delivering the message: epimorphin and mammary epithelial morphogenesis. *Trends Cell Biol.*, 13, 426-434.

Sato K., Ebihara T., Adachi E., Kawashima S., Hattori S. and Irie S. (2000) Possible involvement of aminotelopeptide in self-assembly and thermal stability of collagen I as revealed by its removal with proteases. *J. Biol. Chem.*, 275, 25870-25875.

Segawa D., Miura K., Goto T., Ohshima S., Mikami K., Yoneyama K., Shibuya T., Watanabe D., Kataoka E., Yoshino R. and Watanabe S. (2005) Distribution and isoforms of epimorphin in carbon tetrachloride-induced acute liver injury in mice. *J. Gastroenterol. Hepatol.*, 20, 1769-1780.

Shiojiri N. and Sugiyama Y. (2004) Immunolocalization of extracellular matrix components and integrins during mouse liver development. *Hepatology*, 40, 346-355.

Simian M., Hirai Y., Navre M., Werb Z., Lochter A. and Bissell M. J. (2001) The interplay of matrix metalloproteinases, morphogens and growth factors is necessary for branching of mammary epithelial cells. *Development*, 128, 3117-3131.

Stanulović V. S., Kyrmizi I., Kruithof-de Julio M., Hoogenkamp M., Vermeulen J. L., Ruijter J. M., Talianidis I., Hakvoort T. B. and Lamers W. H. (2007) Hepatic HNF4alpha deficiency induces periportal expression of glutamine synthetase and other pericentral enzymes. *Hepatology*, 45, 433-444.

Sugiyama Y., Koike T. and Shiojiri N. (2007) Immunohistochemical analyses of cell-cell interactions during hepatic organoid formation from fetal mouse liver cells cultured in vitro. *Histochem. Cell Biol.*, 128, 521-531.

Watanabe S., Hirose M., Wang X. E., Ikejima K., Oide H., Kitamura T., Takei Y., Miyazaki A. and Sato N. (1998) A novel hepatic stellate (Ito) cell-derived protein, epimorphin, plays a key role in the late stages of liver regeneration. *Biochem. Biophys. Res. Commun.*, 250, 486-490.

Yoshino R., Miura K., Segawa D., Hirai Y., Goto T., Ohshima S., Mikami K., Yoneyama K., Shibuya T., Watanabe D., Kataoka E., Takeuchi S., Endoh A., Sato W. and Watanabe S. (2006) Epimorphin expression and stellate cell status in mouse liver injury. *Hepatol. Res.*, 34, 238-249.

INDEX

B

C

D

E

F

G

H

I

J

K

L

M

Q

R

T

U

V

W

Y

Z